I0817026

GREAT DISCOVERIES IN SCIENCE

Vaccination

Erik Richardson

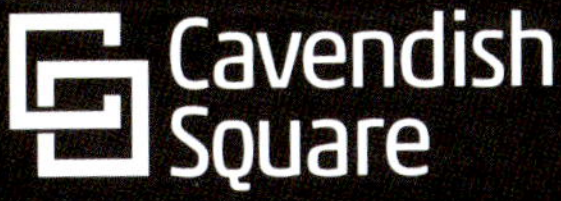

New York

Published in 2018 by Cavendish Square Publishing, LLC
243 5th Avenue, Suite 136, New York, NY 10016

First Edition

CPSIA Compliance Information: Batch #CS17CSQ

All websites were available and accurate when this book was sent to press.

Library of Congress Cataloging-in-Publication Data

Names: Richardson, Erik.
Title: Vaccination / Erik Richardson.
Description: New York : Cavendish Square, 2018. | Series: Great discoveries in science| Includes index.
Identifiers: ISBN 9781502627803 (library bound) | ISBN 9781502627810 (ebook)
Subjects: LCSH: Vaccines--Juvenile literature. | Vaccination--Juvenile literature.
Classification: LCC RA638.R534 2018 | DDC 614.4'7--dc23

Editorial Director: David McNamara
Editor: Caitlyn Miller
Copy Editor: Michele Suchomel-Casey
Associate Art Director: Amy Greenan
Designer: Lindsey Auten
Production Coordinator: Karol Szymczuk
Photo Research: J8 Media

The photographs in this book are used by permission and through the courtesy of: Cover AB Still Ltd/Getty Images; p. 4 plenoy m/Shutterstock.com; p. 8 JacquesLouis David/Wikimedia Commons/File:Jacques Louis David Bonaparte franchissant le Grand SaintBernard, 20 mai 1800 Google Art Project.jpg; p. 11 Universal History Archive/UIG via Getty Images; p. 12 Ann Ronan Pictures/Print Collector/Getty Images; p. 13 Everett Historical/Shutterstock.com; p. 14 Encyclopaedia Britannica/UIG/Getty Images; p. 15 khlungcenter/Shutterstock.com; p. 17 Bettmann/Getty Images; p. 19 Daily Herald Archive/SSPL/Getty Images; p. 26 Repina Valeriya/Shutterstock.com; p. 29 Wellcome Images/Wikimedia Commons/File:Engraving; 'portrait' of Galen, head and Wellcome L0005549.jpg/CC BY 4.0; p. 30 Kean Collection/Getty Images; p. 32 Hulton Archive/Getty Images; p. 43 Wenceslaus Hollar/Wikimedia Commons/File:Wenceslas Hollar Paracelsus (State 2).jpg/CC SA; p. 44 Wellcome Images/Wikimedia Commons/File:Edward Jenner. Pastel by John Raphael Smith. Wellcome L0026138.jpg/CC BY 4.0; p. 47 Sir Joshua Reynolds/Wikimedia Commons/File:Mary Stuart (17181794), Countess of Bute, after Sir Joshua Reynolds.jpg; p. 50 Wellcome Images/Wikimedia Commons/File:Louis Pasteur (1822 1895), microbiologist and chemist Wellcome M0005223.jpg/CC BY 4.0; p. 52 ullstein bild/ullstein bild via Getty Images; p. 55 United States Army/Wikimedia Commons/File:Walter Reed National Military Medical Center.jpg; p. 58 Bettmann/Getty Images; p. 60 EsHanPhot/Shutterstock.com; p. 65 Wellcome Images/Wikimedia Commons/File:Edward Jenner vaccinating a boy. Oil painting by E.E. Hille Wellcome L0029093.jpg/CC BY 4.0; p. 67 Everett Historical/Shutterstock.com; p. 76 Komsan Loonprom/Shutterstock.com; p. 79 Tkarcher/Wikimedia Commons/File:Herd immunity.svg/CC BY 4.0; p. 83 Encyclopaedia Britannica/UIG Via Getty Images; p. 84 Scott Brinegar/Disney Parks via Getty Images; p. 87 phichet chaiyabin/Shutterstock.com; p. 89 Petty Officer 1st Class Brian A. Goyak/Wikimedia Commons/File:Defense.gov photo essay 080324-N-0577G-016.jpg; p. 94 CDC/Charles Farmer/Wikimedia Commons/File:Polio physical therapy.jpg; p. 97 DFID - UK Department for International Development/Wikimedia Commons/File:Preparing a measles vaccine in Ethiopia.jpg; p. 99 SHAUN CURRY/AFP/Getty Images; p. 101 NIAID/Wikimedia Commons/File:Human B Lymphocyte - NIAID.jpg.

Printed in the United States of America

Contents

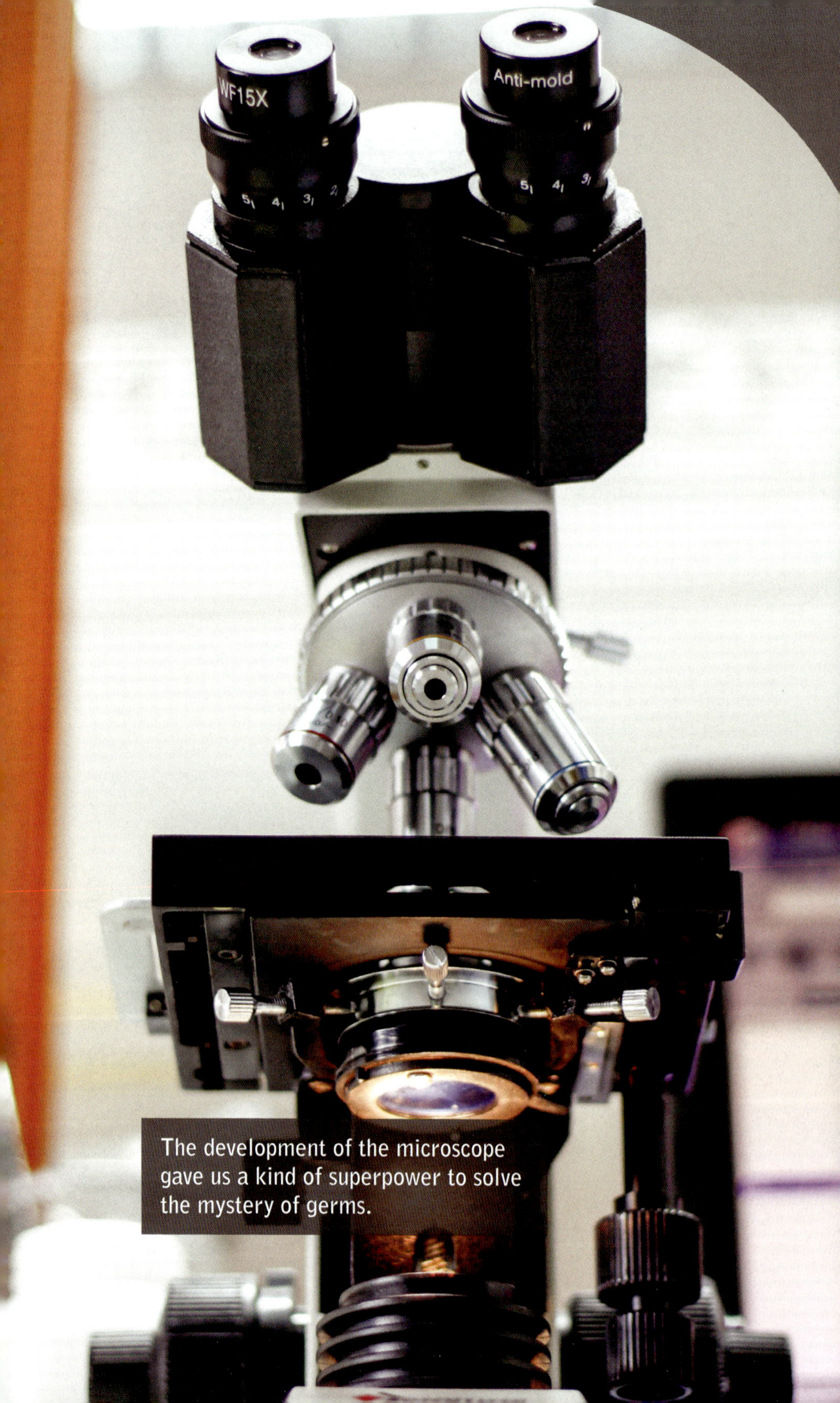

The development of the microscope gave us a kind of superpower to solve the mystery of germs.

Introduction: Waging War on Disease

Some of the deadliest wars in history are not like regular wars. Instead, these wars are fought against opponents so tiny they are not even visible to the human eye, and many of them are not even visible through a normal microscope. Yet, in spite of their tiny size, these invisible armies have killed more people than all the wars waged by mankind put together.

Over the course of this book, we will look at how much damage some of these "armies" of **microbes** have done and how they keep coming back over time to kill people again and again. The story of vaccination and disease is not all grim and depressing, though. We will also meet some brilliant scientific minds who have helped figure out what these invisible enemies are like and how we can fight back in better and better ways.

In the first chapter, we will look at the different kinds of disease. Since this book is not actually about diseases, but about vaccines, we will focus on the diseases that we have developed vaccines to fight against (or that we think we will be able to develop vaccines for). As it turns out, though, these are most of the deadliest diseases ever uncovered.

In chapter two, we will go back in time to get an understanding of why humans fared so poorly in our war against these diseases before the advent of vaccines. The strange mixture of superstition, made-up ideas, and untested theories from ancient times that counted as "medicine" in the 1700s and 1800s made it difficult for society to make real strides in medical care.

Chapter three is where we will be introduced to some of the great heroes in the fight against the evil germs. We will meet a writer, a fiddle player, the man who saved the wine industry in France, and the guy who married Pablo Picasso's former girlfriend—each one of them bringing their different perspectives to the challenge to outsmart our microscopic enemies.

Chapter four will walk you through the timeline, like a small museum, showing how different discoveries and inventions that combat disease happened over time. This will help us understand the shape of our continued practices and how each next step in the path of progress connects and builds up from the steps that had been taken before.

Finally, chapter five will give us a peek at some of the ideas being worked on at the front lines of the war and will help us see how our continued success involves not just things happening in laboratories or inside our immune systems, but also things happening in amusement parks and schools and courtrooms.

Each year, the worldwide impact of contagious diseases like the ones we will learn about in the chapters ahead adds up to millions of deaths each year, even with the great advances in vaccinations and disease-prevention practices. This will get worse as the world population climbs toward an estimated ten billion people by 2050. Not only does the number of people keep climbing, but how much they travel is rising as well, which means any contagious disease can spread far faster than **epidemics** in earlier eras. For comparison, in the 1950s there were approximately fifty-eight million air passengers per year around the world, but more recent numbers show that has grown to almost two billion per year.

We can see the scale of this increase even by looking at a few potential cases, like strains of **malaria**, HIV, and **tuberculosis**, which seem to be evolving around our current solutions. By 2050, these three alone could result in ten million additional deaths per year, and the costs would be almost $100 trillion.

What is more, experts working with research from the World Health Organization and the National Science Foundation estimate that we could be confronted with as many as five new diseases emerging every year as we move forward. A key to success in keeping up with this evolving battle is to find solutions to these emergent diseases as quickly as possible. The earlier we can intervene with an effective vaccine, the lower the impact—not only in lives, but also in costs.

With that little glimpse into the future in mind, let us now turn and explore the history of progress that has led to the point where we are winning the battle against many of these diseases.

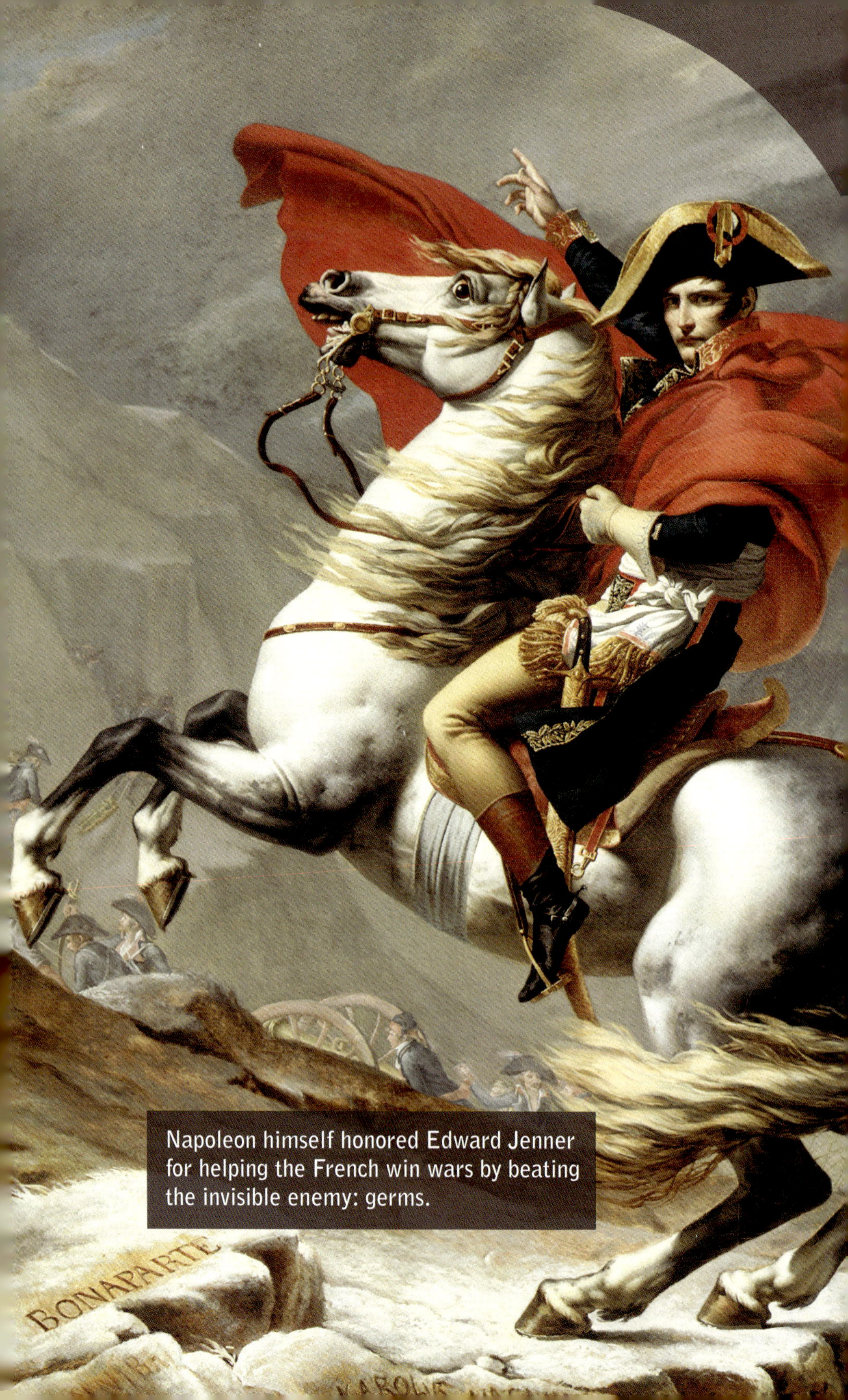

Napoleon himself honored Edward Jenner for helping the French win wars by beating the invisible enemy: germs.

CHAPTER 1

The Problem of Infectious Diseases

To understand the scale of what was accomplished by the great minds whose paths we shall shortly retrace, we must first get a fair glimpse of the size and power of the opponent with which they fought. As we will see, the diseases at hand were more than equal to the greatest armies of the era—for any era. It can be little wonder, then, to see so great a military mind as Napoleon accord the kind of honor to the creator of the first vaccine, Edward Jenner, that would traditionally have been extended to great military heroes. In responding to a request by Jenner, on behalf of the families of prisoners of war, Napoleon responded, "Anything Jenner wants shall be granted. He has been my most faithful servant in the European campaigns." By this, he was referring to the countless number of Napoleon's soldiers who had been saved by the **smallpox** inoculation developed by Jenner. Let us, then, get a sense of the enemy that has come against us again and again.

The ENEMY HORDES CRASHING at OUR GATES

Smallpox

Historians have not been able to pin down precisely the original location from which smallpox began to spread. It might have been Africa, China, or India. It seems to have begun as an animal **virus** that **mutated** and made the jump to the human population. Viruses like this are found in animals in a wide variety of species and ecosystems, and the ability of a mutated animal virus to infect humans is common enough. Smallpox made its way to Europe during the fifth century CE, maybe even shortly before that. Over the course of the Middle Ages, it grew to epidemic scale several times and competed with the bubonic plague as the leading cause of death for long periods.

During the medieval period, it was at the top of the list for causes of death for hundreds of years. The **fatality** rate for those who caught smallpox ranged between 20 percent and 60 percent. The death rate among the elderly was higher because of weakened immunity, and among infants who contracted the disease, fatality could be close to 80 percent.

This was neither its first nor its last impact on the stage of history, though. There was an epidemic around the year 165 CE that coincided with the final era of the Roman Empire; estimates place the death toll around seven million. Smallpox also spread when Muslim and Arabic peoples launched wars of conquest into Europe in the seventh and eighth centuries and due to the Christian Crusades. Once Europeans turned toward conquest in the New World, the disease had become truly worldwide in its reach.

As Christopher Columbus and other European explorers, treasure hunters, and merchants ventured out, Europe was riddled with not just smallpox, but with epidemics of **diphtheria**, influenza, **measles**, even plague. While these diseases wrought havoc in the cities of Europe, in that period killing around 20 percent of the population, the damage was even worse when it came to the Americas.

From its first appearance in 1518 in Hispaniola, smallpox quickly reached other islands like Cuba and Puerto Rico and from there was carried to Mexico. At that point, it was able to spread along trade routes going both north and south. As with the damage to the Roman Empire, so too smallpox played a

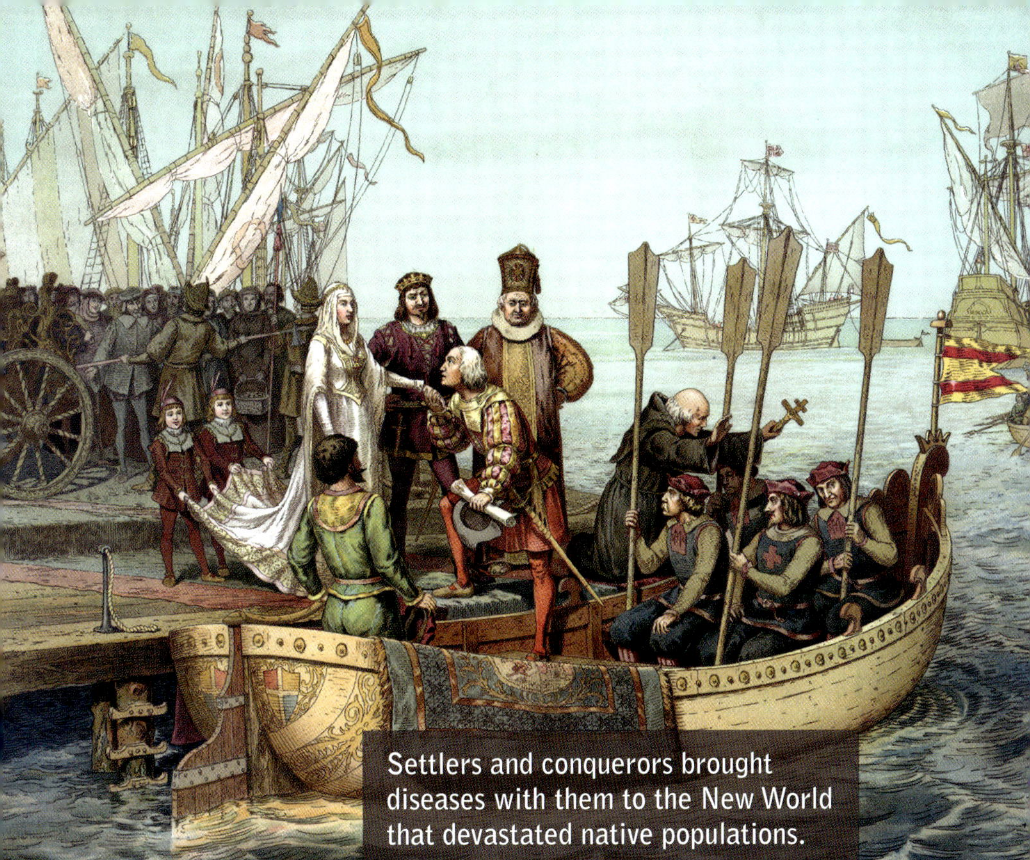
Settlers and conquerors brought diseases with them to the New World that devastated native populations.

role in the fall of the great empires of the Americas, like the Aztecs and the Incas.

While Spanish conquistador Hernán Cortés's group of six hundred was vastly outnumbered in 1519 at first contact, the Aztec numbers—both their warriors and their civilians—had been decimated so he could easily conquer them. It was not smallpox alone, but that was the leader of the diseases the Europeans had brought. The native population of Mexico is estimated to have gone from around twenty million to between one and two million by 1618.

The disease then traveled south doing similar damage. Only a few years after the conquistadors landed in South America, smallpox had wiped out between 60 percent and 85 percent of the population. If not for the destruction from these diseases, including measles and influenza, the small army of two hundred that Spaniard Francisco Pizarro had brought

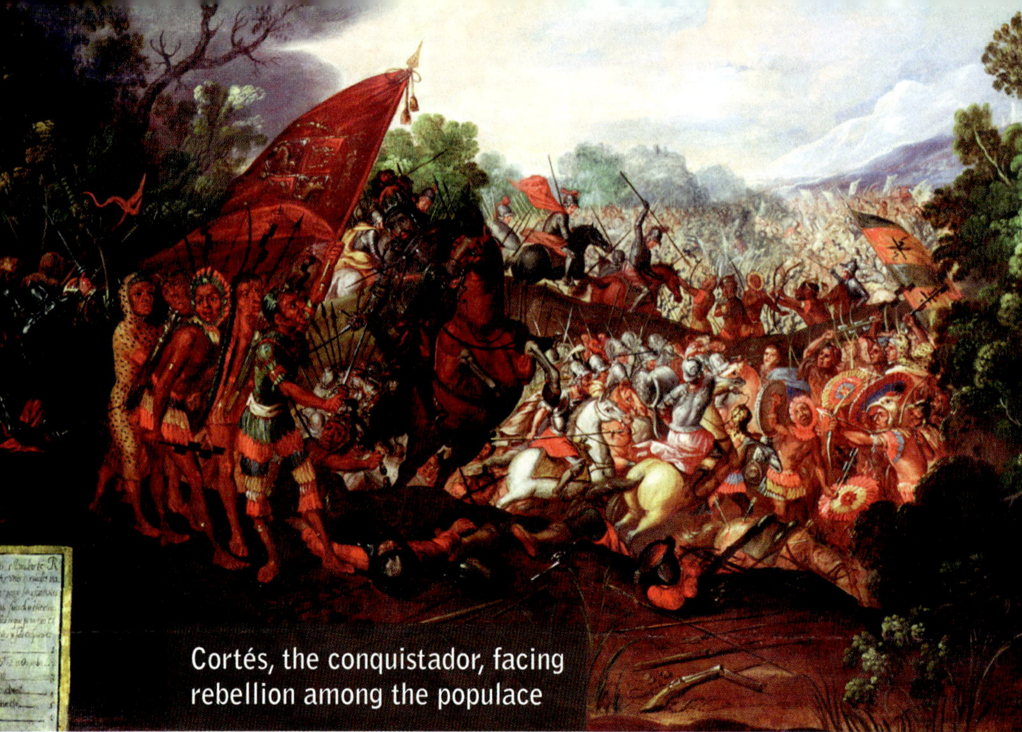
Cortés, the conquistador, facing rebellion among the populace

along would never have been able to make the Incas into slaves as they did.

The story goes very much the same for outsiders arriving to the east coast of America and making first contact with Native Americans in North America. An estimated one and a half million Native Americans died from European diseases in the seventeenth and eighteenth centuries. Often whole villages were wiped out.

By the early nineteenth century, it is thought that as much as 90 percent of the native populations of the New World had been erased by **infections** of Europe. We should not get the impression that the diseases had sailed for the New World like pilgrims, though, for they also continued to wreak havoc back home.

Among those falling to these killers who favor no class were Queen Mary II of England, Tsar Peter II of Russia, and King Louis XV in France. In a move that no force of empire had ever managed, smallpox wiped out eleven different members of the Habsburg dynasty in Austria. There can be little doubt about the profound impact each of these deaths had on the shape of history.

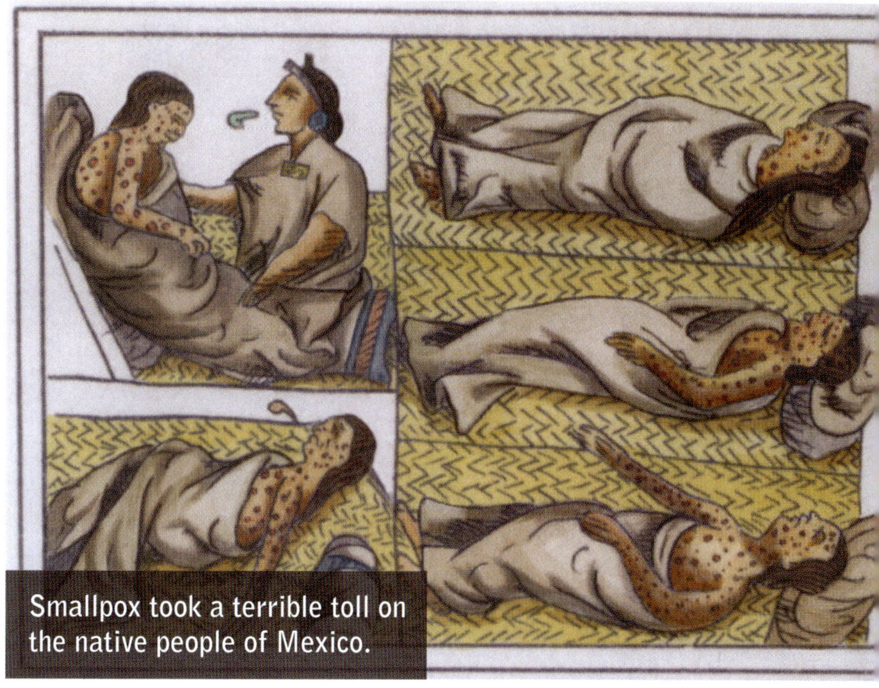
Smallpox took a terrible toll on the native people of Mexico.

Even as late as the twentieth century, and with all the vaccines and the knowledge of modern medicine, it is estimated that almost three hundred million people died from smallpox before it was finally **eradicated**. That number is more than all the deaths from all the wars in the twentieth century (which included both World War I and World War II, remember).

Yellow Fever

Unlike smallpox, we have a pretty clear idea where **yellow fever** originated, and that is from monkeys in the tropical regions of Africa. The virus was then brought over to the Americas—along with the mosquitoes who carry it—as a stowaway on slave ships. It may have been here earlier, but the first **outbreak** recorded is in Barbados in 1647. At that time, Barbados was being run by the English, who were bringing over slaves

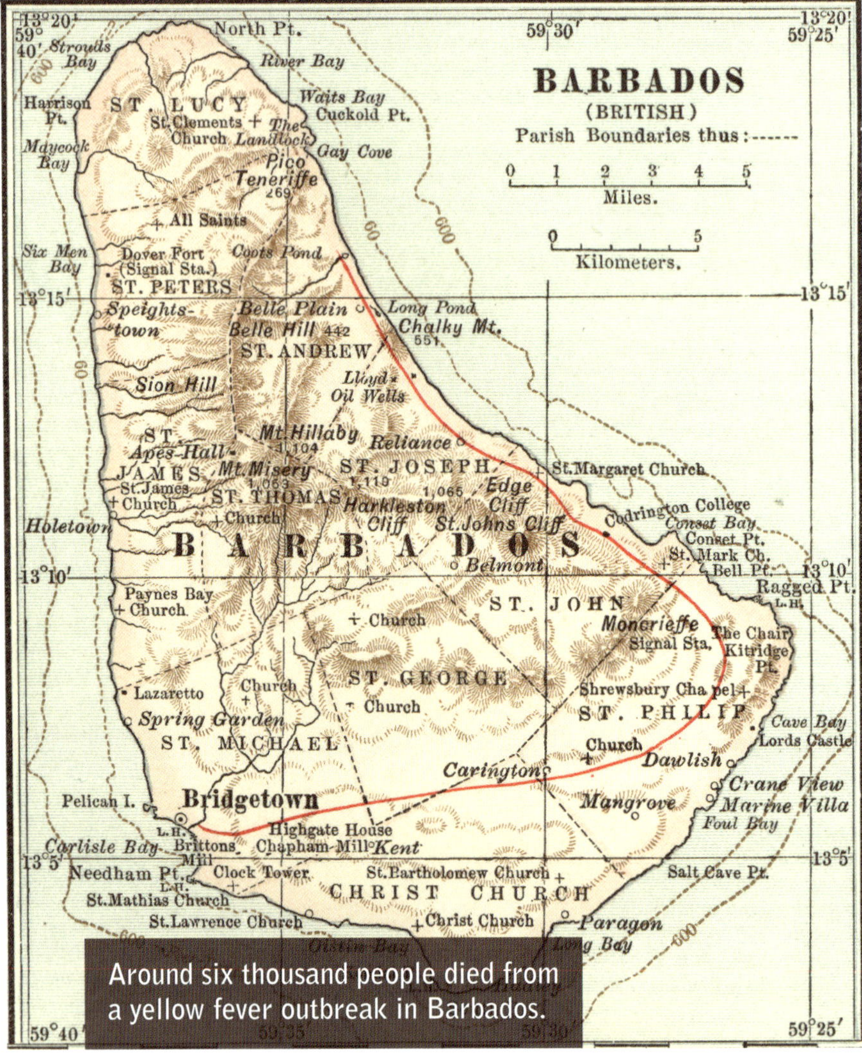

Around six thousand people died from a yellow fever outbreak in Barbados.

for their plantations. Estimates put the death toll around six thousand for this outbreak.

Of course, Barbados was not alone. Port cities around the Caribbean were also hit. It was known as "white man's illness" because it hit the Europeans much harder than it seemed to hit the African slaves. Be that as it may, it quickly spread beyond the port cities to become a problem in the tropical areas, the subtropical regions even, in certain parts of the year, and in areas farther north or south, as long as it warmed up enough for the mosquito population to climb.

As it continued to spread, both overland, as it were, and on ships coming into North America from Africa, yellow fever epidemics swept across parts of the United States again and again during the 1700s and 1800s. When it reached into highly populated cities, the death tolls rose into the thousands.

The first outbreak in the United States was in the late 1690s, but over the next hundred years, outbreaks would rise and fall without clear pattern. In 1793, some refugees trying to escape the epidemic in the Caribbean went to Philadelphia; the disease took hold there, too. By late in the fall, as many as one hundred people were dying from yellow fever every day. In fact, the burden of caring for victims was growing so heavy that the city government was being overwhelmed.

It was only the cold weather coming in that put an end to it. As the mosquitoes dropped off, so did the death rate, although no one saw the connection yet. Port cities remained the focal points for the disease—Charleston, Savannah, Mobile, and New Orleans. Then, in the 1800s, it began spreading up along the Mississippi River Valley. By October 1878, as many as twenty thousand people had died, and the disease had gone as far north as Memphis, Tennessee, killing nearly five thousand residents and driving more than forty-five thousand people to flee the city to wait for the epidemic to pass.

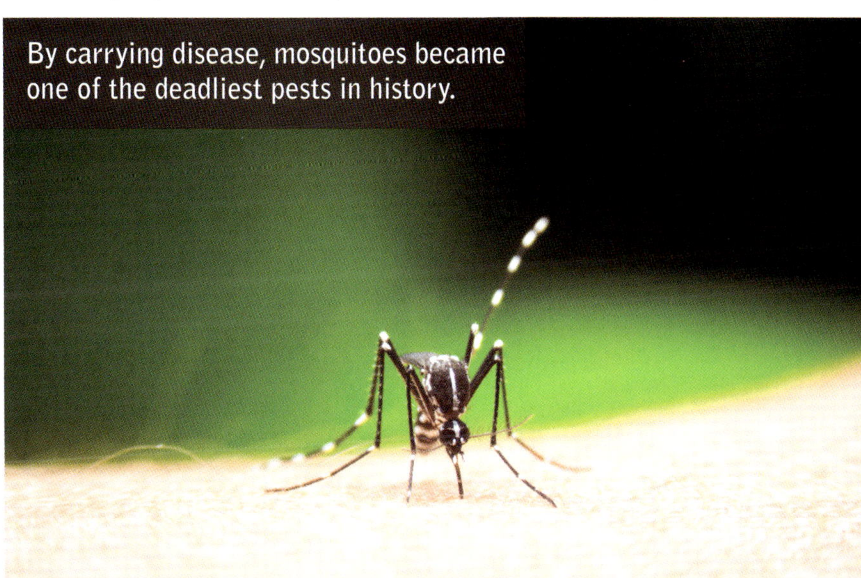

By carrying disease, mosquitoes became one of the deadliest pests in history.

With the last major outbreak being seen in 1905, and the subsequent use of vaccines and techniques to control mosquito populations, yellow fever today is found mainly in certain areas of South America and Africa. Estimates of yearly deaths from yellow fever are still close to thirty thousand because no specific treatment for it, once contracted, has been developed.

Typhoid

Even people who are unfamiliar with typhoid or its impact will often recall the nickname "Typhoid Mary." A cook for families in New York back in the beginning of the twentieth century, Mary Mallon is believed to have actually caused the infection of only fifty people or so, leading to three deaths. The case was sensationalized by the media of the day, though, so it has lasted well beyond its scale.

While typhoid was not recognized as a separate disease until around the 1850s, historians looking back can see points of outbreak and impact going back two thousand years and more into history. In fact, some researchers believe that typhoid was responsible for the plague in 430 BCE that killed Pericles, the ruler of Athens, and almost a third of the citizens. In the aftermath, Sparta gained dominance on the Greek peninsula, thereby bringing the Golden Age of Pericles to an end. The Greek writer Thucydides is our primary source for information about the plague, and he himself contracted and recovered from the disease. There are also historians who believe typhoid is the best explanation for the disappearance of the lost colony of Jamestown, Virginia. It is certainly true that typhoid killed more than six thousand early settlers in the years from 1607 to 1624.

Typhoid would also play a role in several of the US wars. In the Civil War, for example, about eighty-one thousand soldiers in the Union army died from typhoid or the dysentery it caused. Because there were more losses of life to typhoid in the

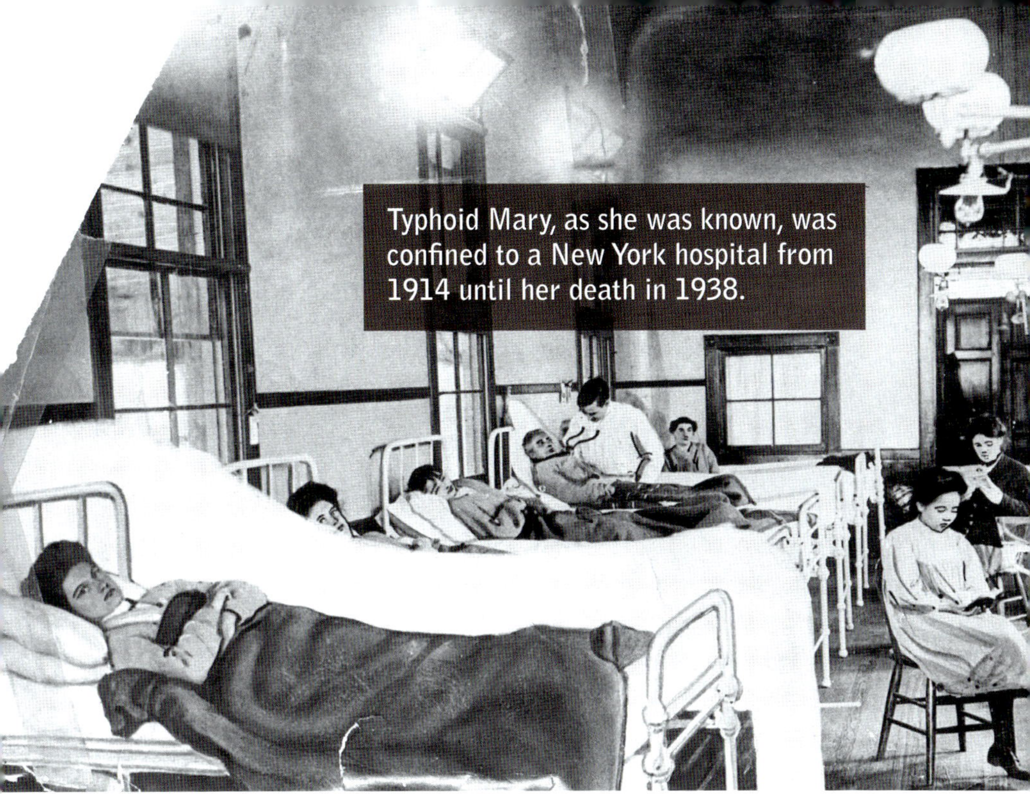

Typhoid Mary, as she was known, was confined to a New York hospital from 1914 until her death in 1938.

Spanish-American War than from yellow fever or from actually being wounded, vaccination was made a requirement for all federal soldiers in 1911.

With use of vaccines and improvements in sanitation issues, like the treatment of drinking water to remove **contamination**, the yearly number of cases of typhoid in industrialized countries is approximately five per million.

Tuberculosis

Evidence of tuberculosis in humans has been found in skeletal remains going back as far as 4000 BCE. Scientists have also found telltale indicators of tuberculosis in Egyptian mummies. In more recent times, tuberculosis began to have an increasing impact from the 1600s on. It reached its peak destruction level during the nineteenth and twentieth centuries and was concentrated in dense city areas. In the years around 1815, tuberculosis was the cause of one in four deaths in England. In

1918, it was still the cause of about one in six deaths in France. At the time it was referred to as "consumption." In addition to coughing up bright red blood, from damage in the lungs, a common side effect was weight loss, so it seemed like the person was being eaten away by the disease.

Polio

Poliomyelitis (commonly shortened to "**polio**") actually represents three different types of related viruses that infect the nervous system, destroying particular kinds of nerve cells and causing paralysis in different parts of the body and even death.

There is evidence that this disease has been around for centuries, but there seem to have been no widespread epidemics prior to the middle and end of the 1800s. From 1841 on, there were a few outbreaks in the United States and Europe. Then, in 1907, there was an explosion of cases in New York where 2,400 people died and thousands more were left with permanent disabilities. Yet another outbreak hit New York in 1916. From that point on, there seemed to be major spikes in cases almost every summer. By the 1940s and 1950s, these epidemics resulted in cases into the five figures; hundreds were killed or paralyzed. Meanwhile, outbreaks were happening in countries like England and Canada, too.

The biggest epidemic on record in the United States came in the summer of 1952. That year there were almost fifty-eight thousand cases reported. Of those, over three thousand people died, and more than twenty-one thousand people were left paralyzed. By that point, the only thing people were more scared of than polio was the atomic bomb.

This was the era that saw the development of the iron lung, a massive chamber that a person would lie inside, with his or her head and neck sticking out. The pressurized compartment could work the lungs if the respiratory muscles had been paralyzed from polio. Iron lungs look rather scary, but they

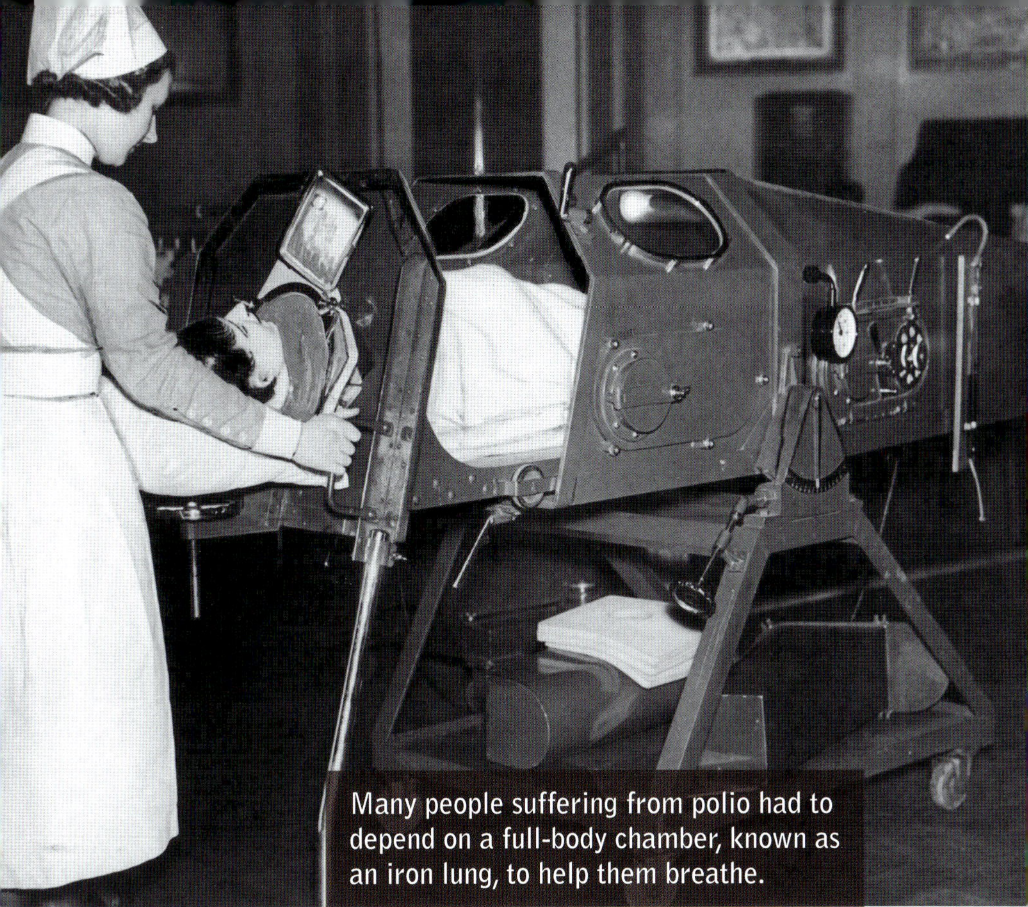

Many people suffering from polio had to depend on a full-body chamber, known as an iron lung, to help them breathe.

saved the lives of a lot of people who were able to finally recover and breathe on their own.

While polio has been targeted for eradication, like smallpox, efforts are stalled by ongoing wars in different susceptible regions—especially Afghanistan and Pakistan. In some affected places, there are rumors that the vaccine can cause HIV or make you sterile, and such rumors make people resistant to get vaccinated, thus perpetuating the spread of disease.

Measles

The last disease we will touch on in this chapter is measles. While some once thought measles might be the underlying disease in the Antonine Plague at the end of the Roman Empire, that theory has fallen out of favor. The first careful description of the disease comes to us from Rhazes, a Persian physician living from 860 to 932 BCE. In his book, *The Book of Smallpox and Measles*, he distinguishes between measles, smallpox, and chickenpox.

In looking at the damage it has done, we find a measles epidemic in Cuba in 1529 that killed almost two-thirds of the natives who had just survived smallpox. By 1531, the disease had contributed to the destruction of native cultures like the Aztecs and the Incas. In the period from 1855 to 2005, it is estimated to have killed almost two hundred million people around the world. In the 1850s in wiped out 20 percent of Hawaii's population. Then, in 1875, measles hit Fiji, killing over forty thousand. That was about one out of every three people!

OTHER KEY MOMENTS along the TIMELINE of OUTBREAKS

To get a better sense of the ongoing struggle against infectious disease, it is helpful not merely to look at each disease separately, but to lay out the epidemics and **pandemics** in historical order. That allows us to appreciate the frequency and impact overall.

In 1545 smallpox, introduced by the Portuguese, was responsible for the deaths of over eight thousand children in Goa, India. More than thirty years later, in 1578, Guillaume de Baillou provided an account of the pertussis epidemic in Paris. Then in 1612, Henry, Prince of Wales died after a short fever. (In 1882, Doctor Norman Moore used descriptions of the illness and notes from the **autopsy** to argue from the evidence that this should be considered the first known English case of typhoid.) In 1613, we have accounts of widespread diphtheria in Spain. It became known as the "year of strangulations." It was called that because obstruction of the throat is often one of the side effects of the disease.

A turning point came in the early 1600s as explorers traveled around the world. By 1625, we see early evidence of smallpox in America. The Jesuits would record that the Indians regarded them with some hostility since they had noticed that natives living closer to Jesuit settlements had higher rates of the disease. Shortly after, in 1633, we see smallpox ravage the pilgrim settlement and the area natives alike. In this outbreak twenty settlers from the *Mayflower* died. Unfortunately, this included their only doctor! In a less-than-shining moment of racism and greed, the governor, John Winthrop, expressed that the death of so many Native Americans was an act of God that cleared the pilgrims' claim to the land they now possessed.

The first medical publication in America in response to a smallpox epidemic running through New England was in 1678. This was a small pamphlet informing people of practices that would (it was believed) help prevent the disease. The epidemic was not, of course, affecting only the settlers. One French courtier, referring to the extreme number of Iroquois who were dying from the disease, referred to it as "the Indian Plague."

In 1694, smallpox in England, which was already rampant and keeping both the doctors and the undertakers overloaded, was responsible for the death of Queen Mary II at the young age of thirty-two. Five years later, yellow fever was so widespread in America that in some cities, like Charleston and Philadelphia, there were few houses without at least one sick person. In 1730, there were heavy losses from smallpox outbreaks in Philadelphia, New York, and Boston. In 1732, yellow fever swept through Charleston, South Carolina, killing people at such a high rate that the town discontinued the normal practice of sounding the church bells when someone died. New York saw a smaller outbreak that same year.

New England faced a diphtheria epidemic in 1735 that took a particularly high toll among children. The overall death rate was 40 percent of those who caught the disease, but it was higher among the young and the elderly, who already have weaker immune systems. Treatment strategies involved making a cut under the tongue (or arm if the tongue was not an option) and applying a honey concoction. This was followed up by salty herbal concoctions and regular enemas.

Then, in 1736, even Benjamin Franklin became an advocate of **variolation**. He lost a son to smallpox and shared his regret in writing so that other parents might not make the mistake he did in not having his son inoculated. Variolation effectiveness was proven again in 1738 when a smallpox outbreak killed almost half of all the Cherokee in the vicinity of Charleston, South Carolina. The fatality rate among white people was 18 percent. The fatality rate was only 4 percent among those who had been inoculated.

In 1775 and 1776, smallpox actually affected the tides of the American Revolution. Boston was suffering from it so that Washington's siege in 1775 was hindered because the occupying British were inoculated, but many of Washington's men had not been. In Quebec, the American force was ten thousand strong, but almost half came down sick with smallpox. John Adams would write to friends that this did more damage than the Canadians, the British, and the Indians all put together.

Yellow fever devastated Philadelphia in 1793, with cases rising over ten thousand and deaths in the thousands. With Philadelphia serving as the state and national capital at the time, both groups of politicians fled the city temporarily. While careful notes about conditions leading up to the outbreak include the observation that the mosquito population was uncommonly high, it would be years yet before they were actually identified as the **vector** for the spread of yellow fever.

The outbreak was bad enough, and suspicions of a connection to sea travelers were strong enough that the city built a small **quarantine** station on an island off the coast. There, travelers would be screened before being allowed to pass through. Those suffering symptoms of yellow fever (and a variety of other illnesses) were assigned to the connecting hospital.

By way of orientation, Edward Jenner's breakthrough—vaccines as we know them—came in 1796. This was the first meaningful counterattack in the long history of the war on infectious disease. In 1800, Dr. Benjamin Waterhouse administered the first vaccinations in the United States to his children. Though efforts to communicate with President Adams had little effect, he then wrote to Vice President Jefferson, who responded very favorably to Waterhouse's project of promoting vaccination.

In 1802, Waterhouse would go on to convince the Massachusetts Board of Health to allow for testing the use of vaccination. When all nineteen volunteers proved that vaccines were a success, the practice began to spread quickly.

The next phase of the war against plague began in 1817 when **cholera** pandemics swept across India and Asia and then spread to the rest of the world. This series of widespread outbreaks falls into several time brackets:

1817–23,

1826–37,

1846–63,

1865–75,

1881–96,

1902–23, and

1961–present.

With the National Vaccine Act of 1840, Britain offered free vaccination for children and, now that it had been replaced by the much safer vaccination, banned variolation. The UK Vaccination Act of 1853 would go on to make infant vaccination mandatory with a consequence of fines and imprisonment for parents who did not comply.

As the last large-scale war before the further development of the germ theory of disease, uncontrolled bacterial infections played a huge role in the American Civil War from 1861 to 1865. Not only did thousands die specifically from measles, but almost two-thirds of all deaths in that war were from infectious diseases. Aside from the deaths, though, the illness itself had a large impact. While only four thousand Union soldiers actually died from measles, for example, there were over sixty-seven thousand cases.

The impact of infectious disease and the role of vaccination was not, of course, confined to the United States and Britain. We see, for instance, that once Germany enacted a vaccination law in 1874, the average yearly deaths in a twelve-year period fell to around two per one hundred thousand people. In contrast, Austria, which did not enact such a law, had yearly average death rates that ranged from around forty to ninety-five per one hundred thousand.

By 1878, yellow fever had continued to grow and spread. The death toll along the Mississippi River Valley had passed thirteen thousand, and John Woolworth, the surgeon general for the Marine Hospital Service, advised the president that it should be dealt with like any other enemy that threatens commerce.

So we have a sense of the scale of damage that has been caused by these various diseases, although they are not the last or only ones we shall meet in this book. We also have a sense of how long they have kept up the attack, coming in waves and alternating in their efforts.

What is more, we have some feel for how there was not only an impact in lives lost at different points along the way, but also for how the whole course of history was shifted—often for the worse. Imagine how different attitudes of conquest and culture might have been if the great civilizations of Central America and South America had pushed back the invaders. The same is true for America itself; how different would things have gone if so many Native Americans had not been erased by the diseases brought by the settlers?

A Closer Look at Rhazes

Abū Bakr Muhammad ibn Zakariyyā al-Rāzī, known as Rhazes (his Latin name), was a brilliant doctor, philosopher, and alchemist who lived in Persia (in an area that would be in modern Iran) from 854 to 925 CE. Rhazes was a man of great learning and wide interests, and he made significant contributions to many different fields.

His greatest contributions were in the area of medicine. He was known as a great medical teacher and an early supporter for using observations and experiments in medicine. Several of his medical books were translated and used by thinkers in the West—including *On Surgery* and *A General Book on Therapy*. His book *al-Judari wa al-Hasbah*, which translates as "On Smallpox and Measles," is considered to be the first scientific project to establish that these were actually two separate diseases instead of being lumped together as one, the way they were before him.

Rhazes also worked to improve the practice of medicine, and he exposed fake doctors, called **charlatans**, who traveled around trying to convince people of the wonderful value of useless treatments and medicines. He deserves particular appreciation for his willingness to hold the ancient Greek doctor Galen accountable, as well, and he was willing to doubt and argue against various conclusions that were often taken as absolute truth. Examples of this include Galen's widely accepted description and treatment of fevers. What is more, Rhazes was critical of the "four humors" theory underneath Galen's approach (and a key aspect of Galen's writing), which we will see continued to misinform medical practice for many centuries after Rhazes.

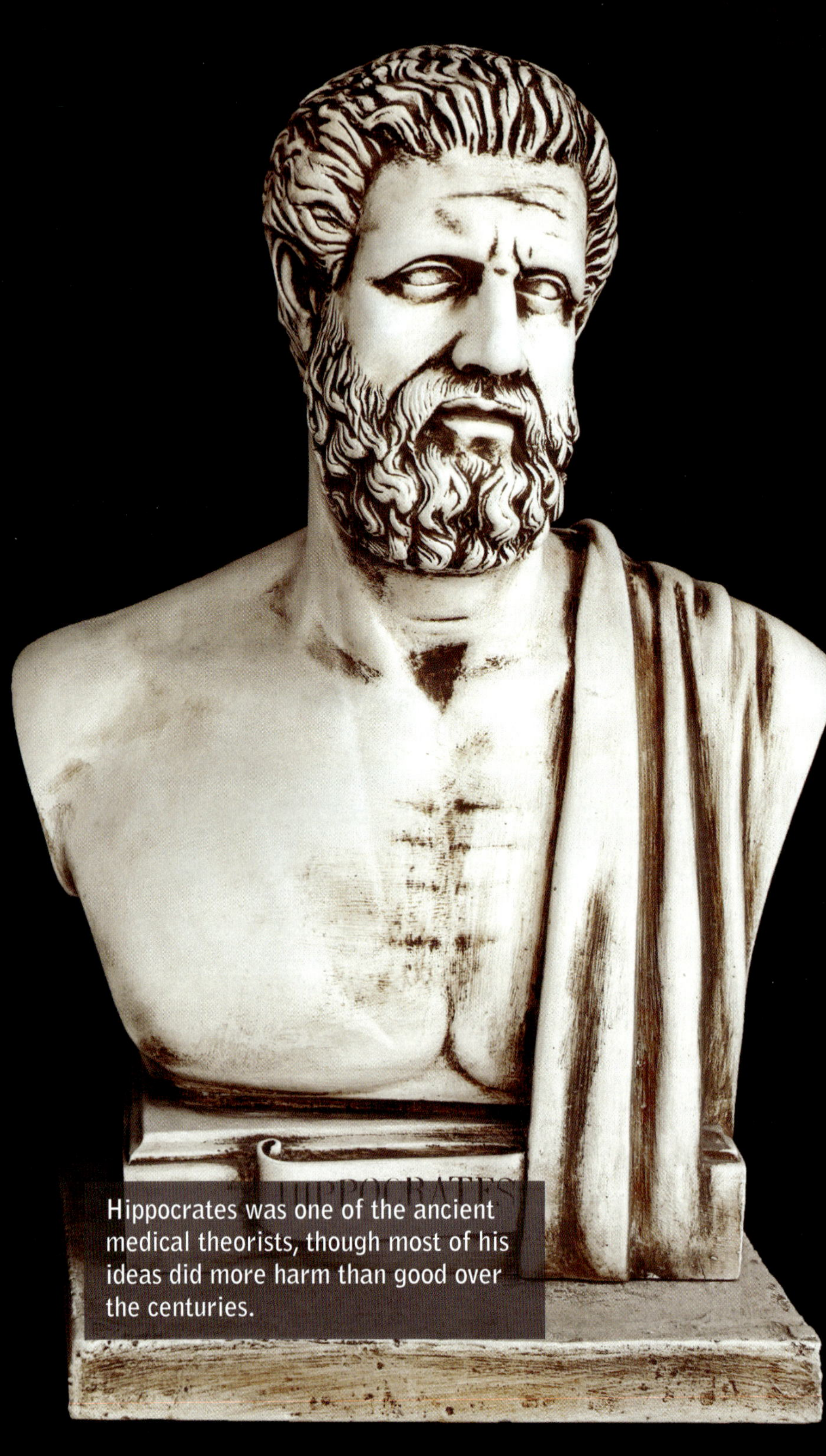

Hippocrates was one of the ancient medical theorists, though most of his ideas did more harm than good over the centuries.

CHAPTER 2

The Science of Battling Contagious Diseases

All through history, humanity has struggled to gain some understanding of the diseases that spark and spread through whole groups like a wildfire. As we saw earlier, these infectious diseases impacted not just lives, but politics, war, and trade as well. Sometimes the theories and the cures were brutal and often hastened the visit from the grim reaper, rather than held him back. In this chapter, we will take a brief tour to see some of the different approaches that were attempted prior to vaccination and other modern methods. We will also take a look at key moments where discoveries and new theories helped move knowledge and treatment forward and lay the groundwork for the modern theory and treatment of infectious diseases.

During our historical tour, we will also see the introduction of one of the large themes that have run through the history of this battle—religion. More specifically we will start to see some of the ways in which religious beliefs repeatedly worked as an obstacle or even sometimes as an active opponent to the medical and scientific worldview in treating the diseases already in motion.

In reading through and seeing this theme, do not jump to the tempting conclusion that all (or even most) religious believers agree with the views that generate this conflict.

There are plenty of faithful in different religions who have a point of view that is compatible with science.

THERE WILL BE BLOOD

Along the entire timeline, and even today, medicine and religion often compete in attempting to own the struggle against sickness. The farther back we go, the more dominant a role religion held in that competition.

Hippocrates, who lived from 460 to 377 BCE, was one of the earliest thinkers to push aside possible supernatural explanations. Instead of disease being caused by the wrath of the gods of Olympus, his book *Airs, Water, and Places* connected illness to features of the water, the soil, climate, and even nutrition. We even get the terms "epidemic" and "endemic" from him. An endemic disease is one that seems to always be around in a population. In contrast, an epidemic is a disease that seems to come and go.

At the same time, what he thought those factors like soil or nutrition did was create an imbalance among the four "fluids" (called humors) of the body. The humors were blood, phlegm, black bile, and yellow bile. Treatment to fix this imbalance meant adding or removing the different fluids from the body. This led to such practices as draining out some of a sick person's blood by various means. Can you imagine being deathly ill and then having blood loss added on top of that?

With Galen, who lived from 131 to 201 CE, we find the theories of earlier thinkers like Hippocrates written down into an organized form. He combined these theories with experiments and with actual dissection of animals to try and understand how anatomy and **physiology** fit into the puzzle. While his work also contained a lot of errors, it would be the standard for more than a thousand years, when Andreas Vesalius (1514–1564) was able to use knowledge from

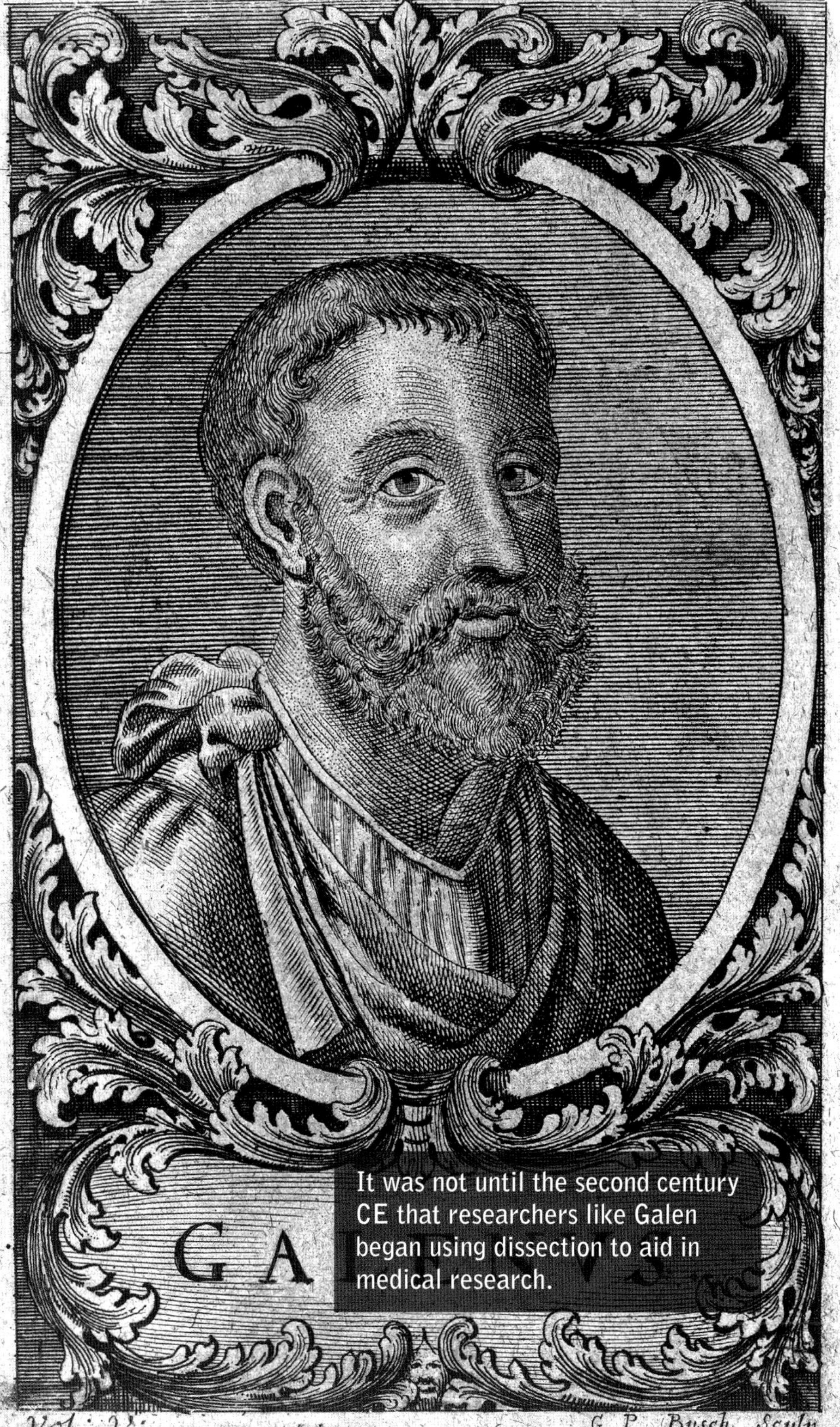

It was not until the second century CE that researchers like Galen began using dissection to aid in medical research.

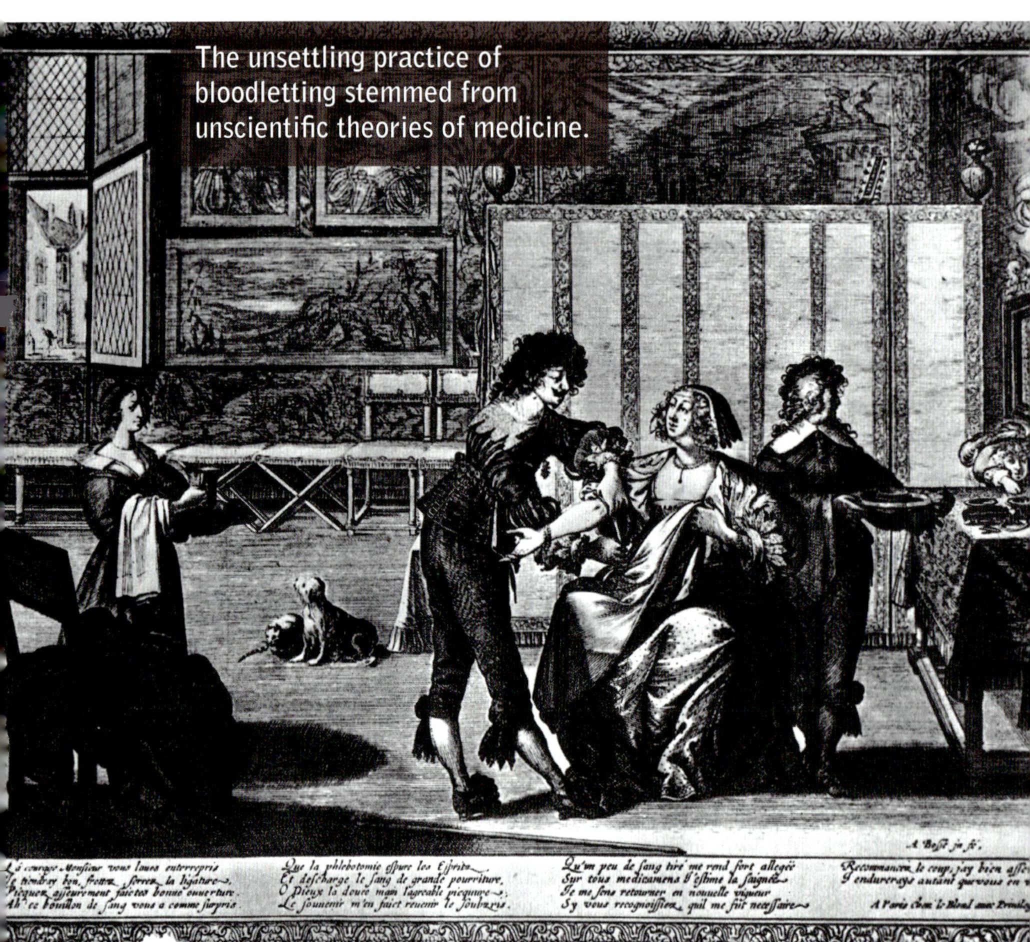

Que la phlebotomie espure les Esprits
Et descharge le sang de grande pourriture,
O Dieux la douce main l'agreable picqueure;
Le souvenir m'en faict revenir le soubzris.
Qu'un peu de sang tiré me rend fort allegée
Sur tous medicamens j'estime la saignée
Je me sens retourner en nouvelle vigueur
Sy vous recognoissiez quil me fût necessaire
The unsettling practice of bloodletting stemmed from unscientific theories of medicine.

dissecting humans to fix a lot of those errors. The central cause of this delay of fifteen centuries was the power of the Christian church and its hardcore opposition to tampering with the bodies of those who had died. Galen was also enthusiastically in favor of theories like bloodletting to rebalance the humors. In fact, when he discovered that both veins and arteries were filled with blood, he built on the theory. Up until then, it was believed that arteries were filled with a kind of air.

Among the wrong-headed ideas that contributed to the theory of bloodletting was the idea that blood did not actually circulate. Instead, they thought that once it was created, it would fulfill its role and then, once used up, it would pool in the extremities. It was sort of like how motor oil needs to be drained from a car every so often and replaced. He then built a complex system to determine which blood (arteries or veins), which side of the body, and which **extremity** was affected by disease based on different symptoms.

Christians connected their faith to this theory determining which holy days and feast days of saints were best for bloodletting. The Middle Ages also saw the practice connected to various theories of horoscopes and astrology. When you think about how the people who survived plagues also had to survive ongoing blood loss, it is a little amazing that more countries didn't just collapse before the Renaissance.

Even as certain kinds of other research were slowly coming along, bloodletting continued to be used. This was done for almost every major disease, including the ones we introduced in chapter one. However, it was also the prescription for things ranging from acne and asthma to the beginning stages of childbirth!

Very early on, people were able to figure out that to control the spread of disease it was important to quarantine the sick and dispose of the bodies of those who died and the possessions of those who had the disease. Unfortunately this had very limited effect, given the many other means

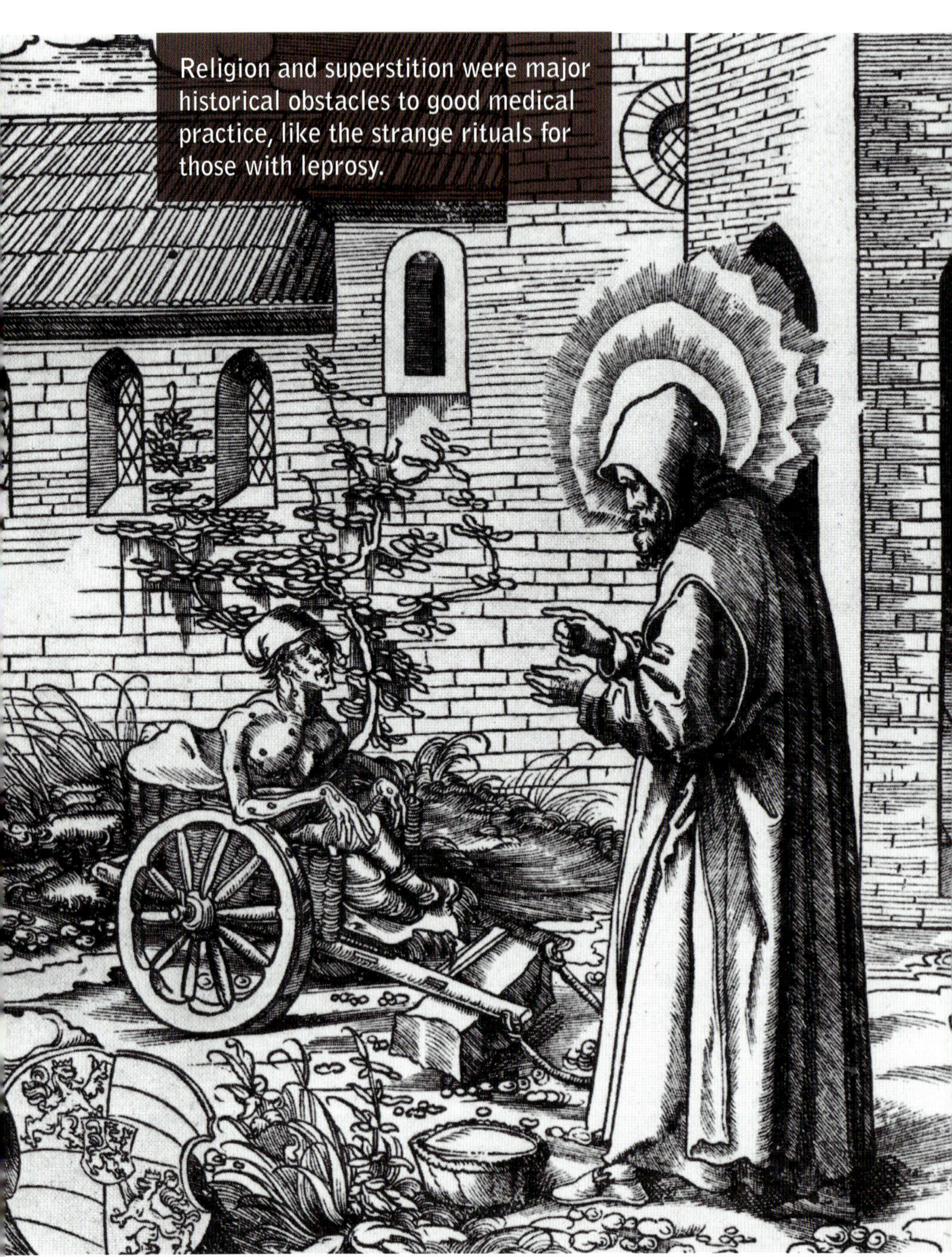

Religion and superstition were major historical obstacles to good medical practice, like the strange rituals for those with leprosy.

of transmission. This was true even before people knew of microbes, as was the case of plague being spread not only by rats, but even by the fleas that had consumed blood from those infected rats.

RITUAL for the "DEAD"

Leprosy was believed all the way back to biblical times to be a result of sinful acts. Certainly people also thought it was contagious, but this was compounded by the fear and **stigmatization** that grew from the religious theories that were added on. Even then, given that the disease is contagious long before the slowly developing symptoms become evident, quarantine probably did very little to control the spread.

By the time we reach the Middle Ages, the theory of sin as the heart of the disease was so powerful that lepers were not only cast out of normal society but reviled. Attitudes switched from mere pity to looking down on them with scorn and contempt. It is here that we find a special religious ceremony called the Mass of Separation. This harsh ceremony included making the leper stand in a grave that had been dug and thereafter considering the person dead. Not only were they never allowed to enter a church but they would not have been able to take communion. While that might or might not sound horrible to you, for those who had strong Catholic faith it would mean additional psychological suffering.

Sometimes we see interesting cases where a thinker might have been partly right, but the idea was still tangled in superstition. A great example of this is an astronomer and doctor named Girolamo Fracastoro, who lived from 1478 to 1553. As explained in his book, *On Contagion, Contagious Diseases, and Their Treatment*, he argued for the idea that diseases were transmitted between people by tiny, invisible particles. He called these *seminaria*, meaning "tiny seeds."

Amazingly, he thought there were separate ones for different diseases and that they made more of themselves once they got inside a person. In his theory, seminaria acted upon the humors of the body.

As part of his theory, he argued that these particles could be passed not only by contact and by things the infected person had touched but could also be transmitted through the air. He was, however, still attached to ancient ideas, and he thought these seeds were affected by the movements of the planets. Epidemics, for example, were caused when certain planets came into alignment.

Since science and religion so often competed, it is a strange irony that during an outbreak of disease, he convinced the pope to move the Council of Trent to a difference city to prevent coming into contact with any contaminated objects.

While we talked about the specific case of leprosy, Christianity invested much more into the unscientific view of medicine. An illuminating example of this was to assign a separate corresponding illness for each of the seven deadly sins. Religious reasoning about the relationship between sin and disease did not only work in one direction. The correct "treatment" was to mount a religious rite or practice. This is reflected in the call for prayer in response to epidemics in colonial America. It is also seen in 1871, when the recovery of the Prince of Wales from typhoid was widely believed to be the result of a nationwide prayer campaign.

This kind of thinking was certainly not limited to the sphere of religion. During the 1600s, for instance, it was widely believed that being touched by the king or queen could heal disease. In this case it was a particular disease, called scrofula, but also known as "the king's evil" because of the healing belief. It was actually tuberculosis that had infected the bones and **lymph glands** and created certain characteristic symptoms. As evidence of how widespread this belief was, consider that just one royal, Charles II, performed nearly ninety thousand such rituals between 1660 and 1682.

It should have broken the theory of disease as punishment for sin to find so many good people also died during epidemics. The fact that it did not presents an interesting contrast with the reasoning we will see shortly in the Henle-Koch postulates for identifying the cause of a disease.

ISOLATING DISEASES and CAUSES

By 1630, well into the Renaissance, we see the use of a kind of tree bark from Peru, called cinchona. It has an active ingredient, quinine, that was used to help treat malaria. It interferes with the growth and reproduction of the microorganisms in the blood.

During this same era of the 1600s, we also see Thomas Sydenham (1624–1689) develop the practice of observing the progress of a patient's symptoms to help classify different kinds of diseases. He outlined his approach and conclusions in the book *Medical Observations*, published in 1676.

Even more extensive work along these lines was done by Giovanni Morgagni (1682–1771). His book, *On the Sites and Causes of Diseases, Investigated by Anatomy*, was published in 1761 when he was seventy-nine. It was the result of over seven hundred autopsies. Here Morgagni matched up specific signs and symptoms to observable effects on the organs and tissues. The approach taken by these two helped lay the groundwork for the future practice of looking for separate specific causes for separate diseases.

During that same period, one of the greatest inventions in history came along and changed the future shape of biology and **epidemiology**. The first great step in this direction was taken by the English scientist Robert Hooke (1635–1703). Among his many scientific discoveries, his work with the microscope is probably his most famous. His book *Micrographia* was published in 1665, and it contained numerous drawings of his different discoveries examining everything from snowflakes to tiny fossils. It helped inspire many others to take up this research tool and help push sciences like biology and epidemiology forward.

One of those other researchers was Anton van Leeuwenhoek, a Dutch scientist who lived from 1632 to 1723. He worked in his spare time to develop better lenses for the recently invented microscope; his design would not be improved until the nineteenth century. With an incredible magnification of 270 times, he was to discover **protozoa** in 1674. This was followed a few years later by the observation of blood cells and actual **bacteria**. Although he had discovered microorganisms, he did not connect them to the cause of diseases. He referred to these tiny organisms as "animalcules."

SEVENTEENTH and EIGHTEENTH CENTURIES

Bloodletting was not the only destructive or wrong-headed medical practice that carried on into the seventeenth and eighteenth centuries. In the seventeenth century, it was believed, for instance, that swallowing a spider would help to reduce a fever and that eating woodlice was a treatment for whooping cough (pertussis). Compared to that, cough medicine is not as bad as it seems!

Although William Harvey, the English researcher, published his work showing that blood circulates, in 1628, the practice of bloodletting was scarcely dampened. It would, however, play a more important role as the development of vaccines unfolded in the later nineteenth century.

Not only were medical uses of plants and minerals infected with a kind of magical thinking, there were even more outright examples of superstition and magic. For instance, to help with the healing of an amputation, the weapon that had caused the wound was brought near and a salve was put on the weapon.

It was believed that this would affect any particles from the weapon that had remained behind in the wound.

As we move on into the eighteenth century, a number of other practices continued to persist. These may have had some placebo effect, when a patient derives benefit from his or her faith in the treatment and not from the treatment itself. While most are less dangerous than bloodletting, in principle, we can recognize the potential negative impact of each practice.

While bloodletting was one of the most extreme examples in many ways, it was closely related to theories that various kinds of **toxins** could be flushed out of the body along with bodily fluids. Surprisingly this same unscientific thinking can be found in modern practices like juice fasts and any number of related dietary practices. We will consider this a little more in chapter five.

Medical practice on into the 1700s and 1800s, then, was more or less dominated by a mixture of practices like the use of enemas to flush out the colon, laxatives to cause extra bowel movements, and administering emetics, which were different chemicals and concoctions that caused vomiting. This theory is also reflected in procedures to cause extreme sweating and even using large amounts of mercury to trigger the body to produce large amounts of saliva. Mercury is, of course, highly poisonous and caused a lot of damaging side effects.

The "draw it out" theory of medical malpractice can also be seen in certain other practices for treating different diseases. One of these is cupping, in which cups were heated and then placed upside down on the person's body so that the vacuum pressure created by the cooling air under the cup could effectively suck out the disease. While this could cause mild burns, akin to sunburn, it was less aggressive than the practice of blistering.

In blistering, a fine ground substance, often from the carapace of certain beetles, was mixed into a paste and applied to the skin to cause extreme blisters to form. Other possible substances included pepper and mustard seed. (This is eerily similar to the World War I use of mustard gas to cause damaging blisters.) Once the blisters had drawn fluid out of the body along with the disease-causing toxins, the blisters would be drained and treated with ointment to heal.

It can be a little hard to read about some of these treatments, so let us turn to talk about a different part of pre-vaccine thinking about disease. This theory will hurt less but probably stink more.

MIASMA THEORY

The **miasma** theory for the cause of disease originated in the Middle Ages and survived all the way into the mid-1800s. In this model, foul-smelling air contained a kind of poisonous vapor that had particles of decomposing matter, which is what made it smell foul. The name for malaria, which killed so many, was actually based on this theory. The word comes from combining the Italian words for "bad" (*mala*) and "air" (*aria*).

Miasma was also referred to as "night air," which relates to various odd theories about making sure windows were closed at night for certain kinds of illnesses (above and beyond it being harmful because of its cool temperature). It was also common practice for anyone who was weak (like children or the elderly) to stay indoors after dark.

It might seem silly for people in England in the nineteenth century to still believe this, but if we consider the evidence in its favor, we can understand their thinking. Because of the way the Industrial Revolution swept through England, quickly squeezing people into cities, a lot of the poor, smelly areas of the city were also where epidemics seemed to break out. As it happened, the things they did to try and improve those conditions, like better sanitation and improved housing, cut down on the growth and spread of bacteria by accident. That means the efforts actually helped reduce the disease levels, even though not for the reason they thought.

GERM THEORY of DISEASE

Some of those trends in isolating diseases and causes will carry forward to overlap and interact with the development of vaccines proper. One of those is the development of the germ theory of disease, which came to replace the miasma theory.

In addition to the forward-looking theory of Fracastoro, there was also important work done by an Italian **entomologist** named Agostino Bassi (1773–1856). In his research on insects, he discovered that a particular disease in silkworms, called muscardine, was caused by a small parasitic fungus. In a strange kind of fame, the fungus was named after him: *Beauveria bassiana*. He went on to argue, in 1844, that this was the mechanism not only of bug diseases, but of diseases in plants, animals, and humans as well. His examples included measles and the plague, though he was not able to establish the strong scientific proof for his theory.

Bassi would go on to produce research on cholera and leprosy, as well as related subjects in cheese and winemaking (both are connected with bacteria and fermentation). We can appreciate how much of an influence he was by considering that Louis Pasteur, who invented the process of pasteurization, kept a picture of Bassi in his office.

Friedrich Gustav Jacob Henle was a German scientist and doctor who lived from 1809 to 1885. In addition to significant developments in anatomy, he is also credited as one of the early modern proponents of the germ theory of disease. His essay, called "On Miasma and Contagions," was published in 1840. This followed in the footsteps of Girolamo Fracastoro and Agostino Bassi.

Henle's student Robert Koch would go on to succeed in finding the specific species of bacteria that caused cholera and tuberculosis, but his strategy in isolating it was built on work by Henle. Thus, the requirements for defining the correct disease-causing **pathogens** are known as the Henle-Koch postulates.

Henle-Koch Postulates

Although modern research of further kinds of pathogens has led to replacing the Henle-Koch postulates, they were vital to the development of vaccines. The rules are:

1. The microorganism must be found in abundance in all organisms suffering from the disease but should not be found in healthy organisms.

2. The microorganism must be isolated from a diseased organism and grown in pure culture.

3. The cultured microorganism should cause disease when introduced into a healthy organism.

4. The microorganism must be re-isolated from the inoculated, diseased experimental host and identified as being identical to the original specific causative agent.

In fairness, Koch himself found cases where the rules did not apply quite so rigidly as they sound. As one example, he was familiar with cases like the cholera-causing bacteria, which can be found in healthy people as well as sick ones (so it breaks rule number one). We should appreciate the kind of reasoning that is built into this set of requirements, even if the specific requirements have become outdated. Earlier thinkers like Sydenham and Morgagni would have seen Henle-Koch postulates as a continuation of the same logic they had tried to bring to the practice of medicine.

VARIOLATION

In chapter three we will step to the side, so to speak, and meet some of the brilliant, inventive minds we have mentioned already and a number whom we have not yet talked about. In chapter four we will take up the timeline of the war on disease. In that regard, there is one practice that should be introduced here, even though it will be discusses further in chapter four: the practice of variolation.

Variolation is an old method for immunizing people against smallpox by using some matter—often tissue or scabs—to infect them with the disease. This practice usually resulted in a less destructive case of the disease, which gave the patient's body a chance to build up its defensive ability before full-blown contact. We might think of this as a warm-up round for our immune systems.

The method had been practiced in places like India and China for centuries before the West became aware of it. An important woman named Lady Montagu learned of it through visiting with Turkish ladies while she was living in Istanbul, and Cotton Mather, the colonial clergyman, learned about it from one of his slaves. In deciding where to include the topic and how to treat it, a couple of things must be kept in mind: Lady Montagu is the only nonscientist in the catalog of heroes in this book. Also, variolation was not quite yet what we would call science, since there was no real understanding of its causes or reasons for working. While such time-tested practices are a foundation for science, they are, themselves, something like a craft.

Paracelsus and the Quest for Science-Based Medicine

Paracelsus was the common name of Philippus Aureolus Theophrastus Bombasus von Hohenheim, a German-Swiss physician and alchemist who lived from 1493 to 1541. Among his contributions was the 1530 book *Der Grossen Wundartzney* ("Great Surgery Book").

He grew up in a village in southern Austria and attended the school where his father taught chemistry. Students there were trained for careers in mining operations, so he learned a great deal about chemistry and **metallurgy**. He then went on to study for a time at various universities. He finished his bachelor's degree in medicine in 1510 from the University of Vienna and went on to earn a doctoral degree from the University of Ferrara in 1515. Paracelsus then spent the next few years traveling around Europe, with a variety of adventures (and misadventures), all the while learning what he could about **alchemy**.

When he finally returned home, his fame and his many amazing medical cures had reached home ahead of him. He was offered a position as town doctor and as a professor of medicine in Basel, Switzerland. Students from all over Europe flocked to hear his lectures. Like Rhazes, he worked to deflate quack practices of many doctors of his time.

At the heart of his contributions to medicine was his effort to replace many crackpot procedures using herbs with those utilizing chemistry and mineral ingredients, like mercury and copper sulfate. While many of his efforts were built on erroneous ideas, he nonetheless opened an entirely new path for the development of medicine.

EFFIGIES PARASELCI MEDICI CELEBERRIMI
Edura fortis Fata refringere
Decoctá callens jura Machaonis
Artesque Phœbæas salubri
Mente PARACELSVS elaborat
Eheu laborans nec tamen irrita
Decreta reddet lucida perbrevi
Mors decolorabit facemque
Purpuream solvet favillas.
P. P. Rub pinxit
P. Stent Excud.
Sould by John Overton at the white horse neere the fountaine

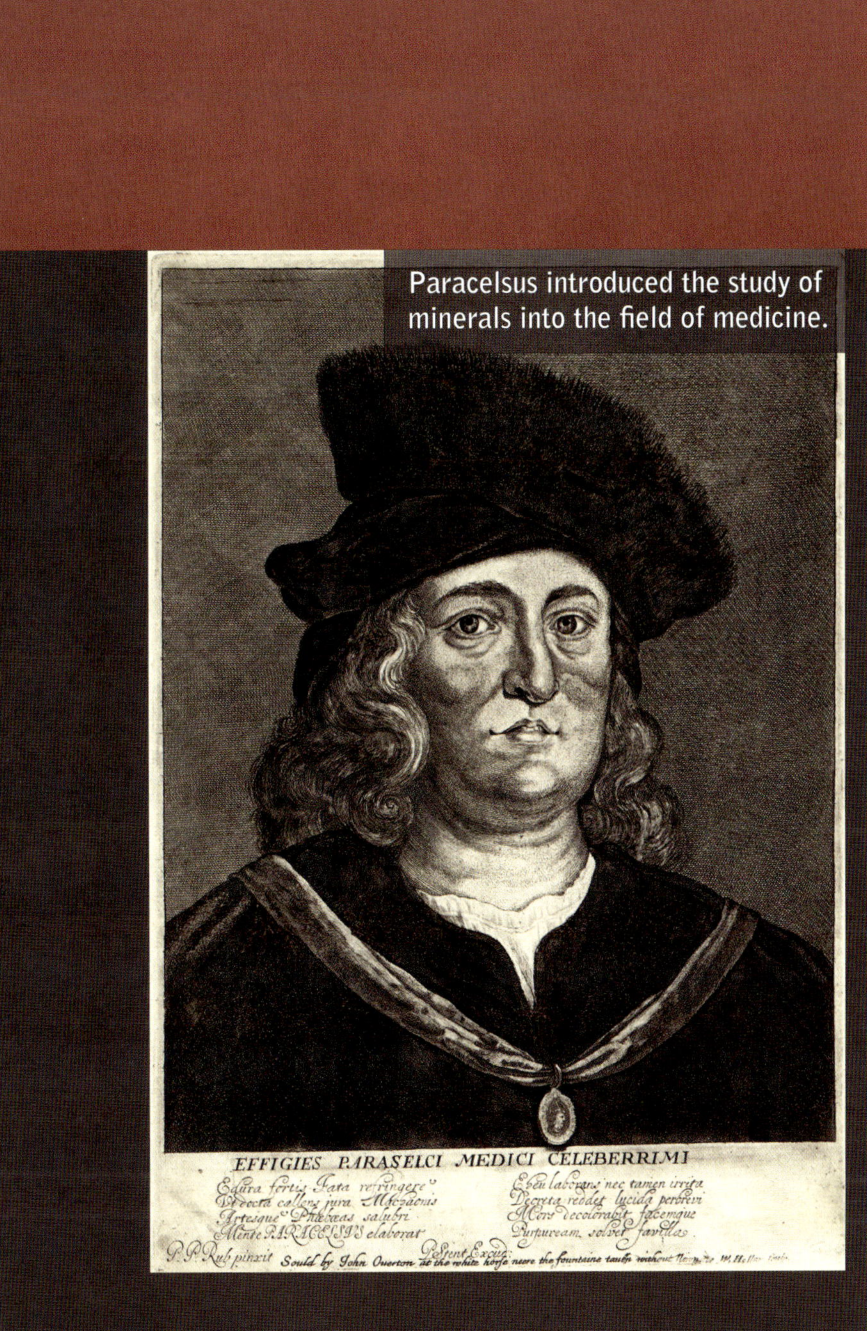

Paracelsus introduced the study of minerals into the field of medicine.

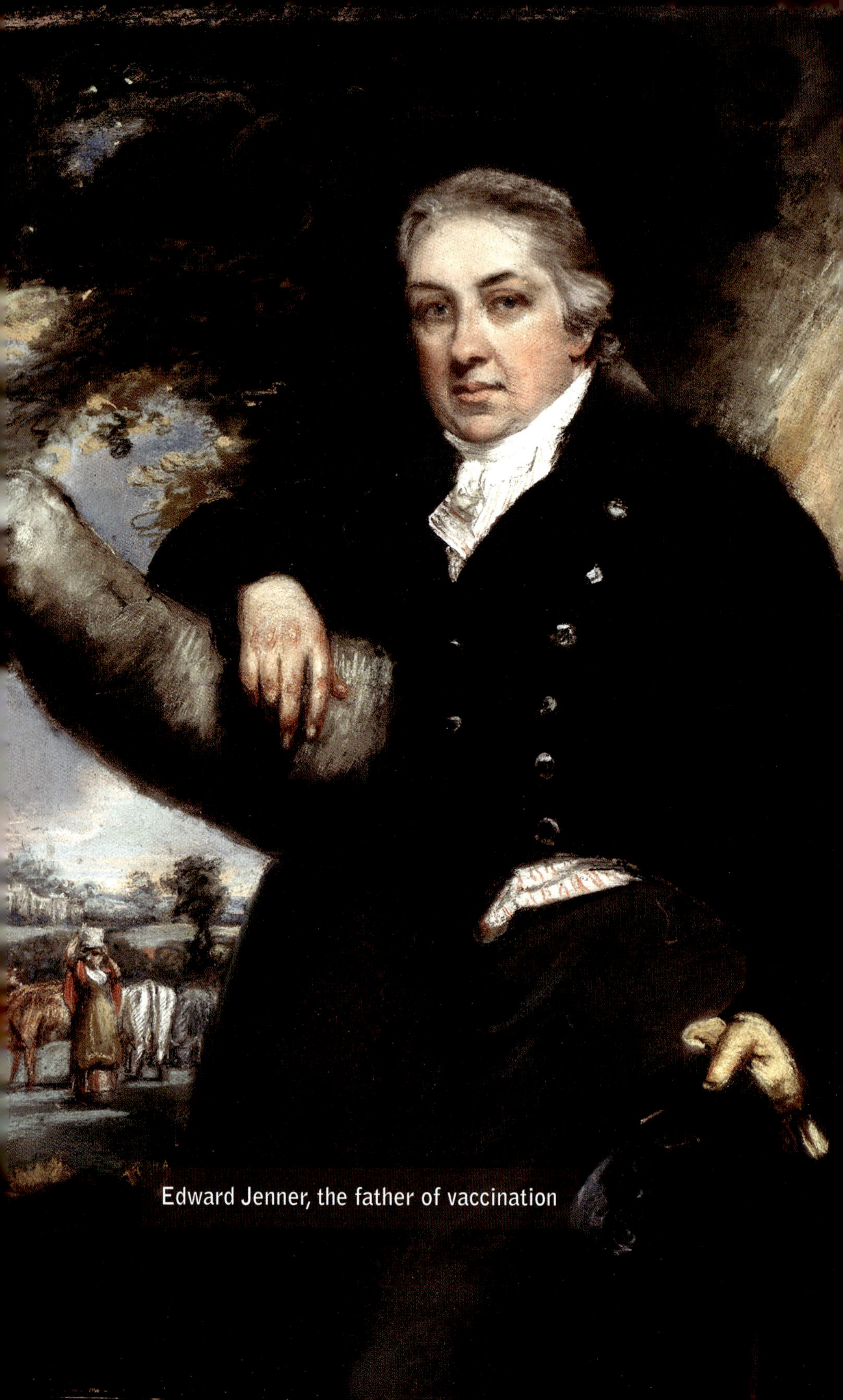

Edward Jenner, the father of vaccination

CHAPTER 3

The Major Players in the Discovery

In the long, slow fight to develop new vaccines for diseases and to get those vaccines into the arms of enough people, and to do it often enough, there are far more heroes than we could hope to cover in one chapter, or even in one book. Rather than attempt to do that, this chapter will try instead to at least introduce some of the most important characters who played a key part along the way.

As you read through the stories and the brief sketches of their lives and work, there are a couple of particularly valuable ideas to hold in mind. The first, and really the most important, is that in spite of how it often seems, these people were not magical. They were just normal people. When they weren't in the lab working to outsmart diseases, they did normal things like drawing, playing the fiddle, arguing with their kids, and so on. That is important because the fight goes on and each of us is capable of becoming one of the central players in the field of science.

The second idea to hold in mind, so it will help you appreciate how they managed to pull off the great achievements, is that there were a thousand small steps they climbed to get to the top of that pyramid (or hill or whatever metaphor you prefer). Louis Pasteur and Jonas Salk did not just wake up one day and think, "Hey, I'll make a ground-breaking, world-changing discovery today." No fairy godmother tapped them with a wand and suddenly filled their head with knowledge about anatomy and biology and germs. They loaded that information in there slowly. They went to college for years and years. Sometimes their projects and their jobs were interesting, sometimes they were routine or unpleasant. They wanted to quit when things went badly or experiments failed or one of their children died. Pasteur didn't suddenly have a vision and see how bacteria worked. He studied fermentation. He worked on smaller problems like why worms were dying. Only then did he have enough little building blocks saved up to build something amazing, like a picture of how **rabies** works.

LADY MARY MONTAGU

Mary Montagu was born Mary Pierrepont in London in 1689. She was the eldest child of the 5th Earl of Kingston and Lady Mary Fielding. It is a funny twist of history that she is most remembered for her important influence on the development of a branch of modern science and in a real sense for saving millions and millions of lives because she was actually a talented writer.

Instead of a marriage her father had arranged for her, she eloped with Edward Wortley Montagu, a member of Parliament with whom she had been corresponding. That was in 1712. Sadly, Mary's younger brother died in 1713 from smallpox, the same year Mary's son was born (also named Edward). Then in 1715, she came down with smallpox as well. Though she survived, her renowned beauty had been marred by the scarring so characteristic of the disease.

In 1716, her husband, Edward, was given the prestigious role of ambassador to Turkey, and they moved to Istanbul (it was still called Constantinople at that point). Her letters based on her time and travels in the region are some of her best writing. It was also during this time that she became familiar with the practice of variolation.

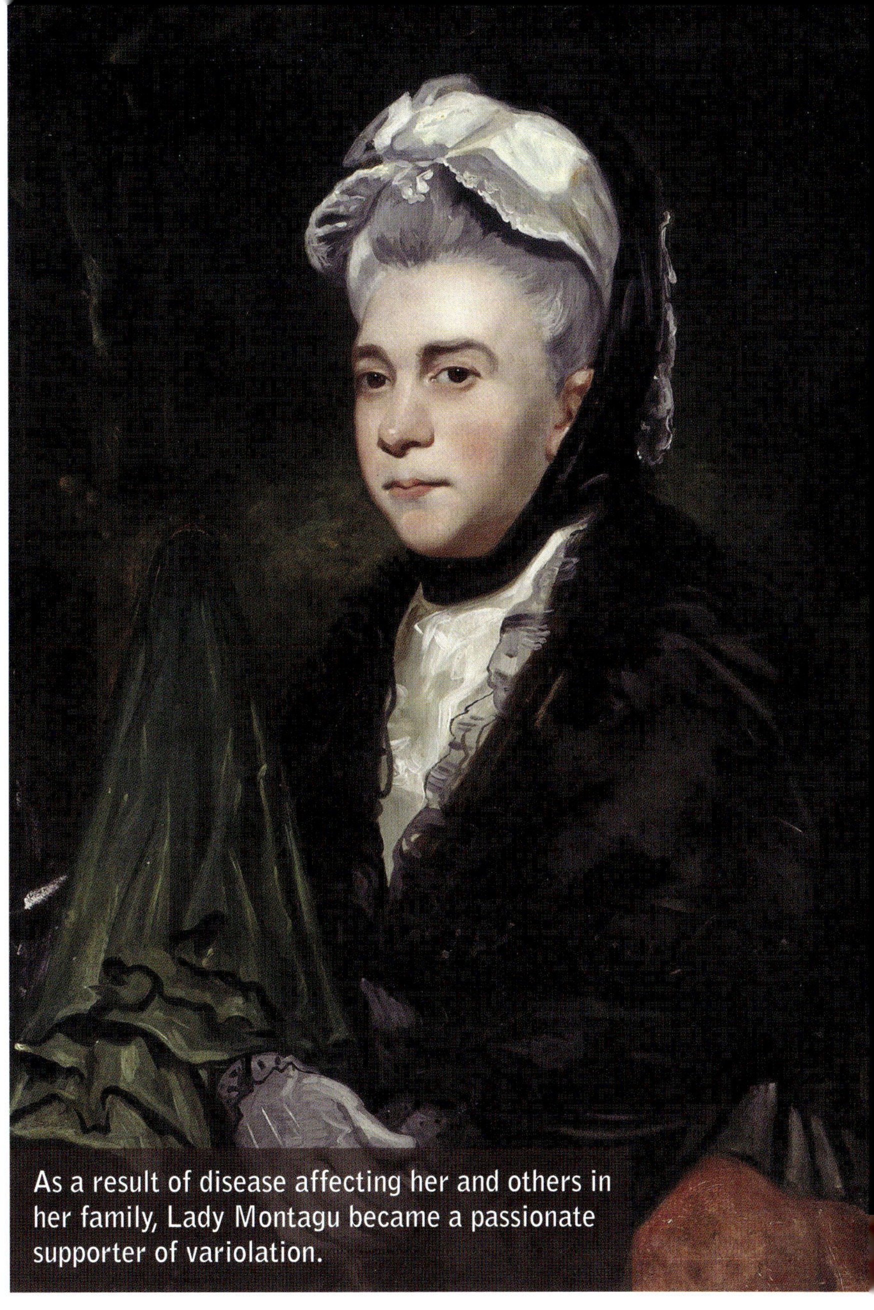
As a result of disease affecting her and others in her family, Lady Montagu became a passionate supporter of variolation.

Her husband's position as ambassador ended in 1718, and during the time before they returned home their second child, Mary, was born. The younger Mary would grow up to marry John Stuart, an earl who served as British prime minister from 1762 to 1763. After returning to England, the elder Mary focused on various writing projects including a correspondence with Alexander Pope and a spirited attack on Jonathan Swift (author of *Gulliver's Travels*).

Later years found her pursuing a couple of different ill-fated affairs and living apart from her husband for a number of years—first in France and then in Venice. After her husband died in 1756, she moved back to England. Though she was reconciled with her daughter (the parents had disapproved of the younger Mary's marriage), London no longer held any interest for Lady Mary, and she would have left again for Italy but fell ill with cancer and died.

EDWARD JENNER

Edward Jenner was born in 1749 in Berkeley, England, and died in 1823. His pioneering work would earn him credit as the father of immunology. He was born into a large family of an Anglican priest. Edward was child number eight (of nine). His father died when he was five, so he was brought up by an older brother, who was a clergyman as well.

At the age of thirteen or fourteen, Jenner became an apprentice to a local surgeon for seven years, and his experience was to have an important influence. In 1770, he traveled to St. George's Hospital in London to become a pupil of John Hunter, one of the top surgeons in London. His learning under Hunter went beyond just basic medical practice to include anatomy and physiology—fields that are normal for doctors to study in our own day and age, but back then it was not so common. Even after Jenner returned to the countryside to be a practicing doctor, the two men would keep up a correspondence for the rest of Hunter's life.

Jenner proved to be a well-rounded man. Not only did he succeed as a country doctor, but he authored a few medical research papers for medical groups, played the violin, and pursued his interests as a naturalist studying things like bird migration. He even published a study on nesting habits of the cuckoo.

He did not marry until 1788, when he was thirty-nine, and the couple had three children, one of whom died of tuberculosis at the age of twenty-one. Jenner was famous for his pioneering work in creating a vaccine for smallpox, including holding the esteem of Napoleon himself, as we saw in the opening pages of the book. This was no idle talk at a time when France was at war with England. In fact, Jenner successfully arranged for Napoleon to release a number of prominent English prisoners of war. In 1815, Jenner's wife passed away from tuberculosis, and he decided to retire.

In his later years, returning home after having given up his medical practice to promote the growth of vaccination, he was elected mayor of Berkeley and continued his interests as a naturalist, including giving a presentation about migration to the Royal Society in 1823—the same year he died.

LOUIS PASTEUR

Louis Pasteur (1822–1895) was a chemist and microbiologist who would stand tall even in the most esteemed company of scientists in history. He was born in Dole, France, where his father was a struggling tanner who had received the Legion of Honor for his service in the Napoleonic Wars. In 1827, Pasteur's family moved to Arbois, and he started school there in 1831. There was little evidence of his great mind at this point, and he was more interested in drawing and fishing than in studying. Nonetheless, he went on to earn a bachelor of arts degree in 1840 and a bachelor of science degree in 1842, both from the Royal College of Besançon.

He entered École Normale Supérieure in 1843. Here he studied chemistry and became a teaching assistant to Jean-Baptiste-André Dumas, a prominent chemist. After finishing his master's degree in 1845, Pasteur earned his doctoral degree in science in 1847 and became a physics teacher at a secondary school. Within a year, he was offered a higher position as

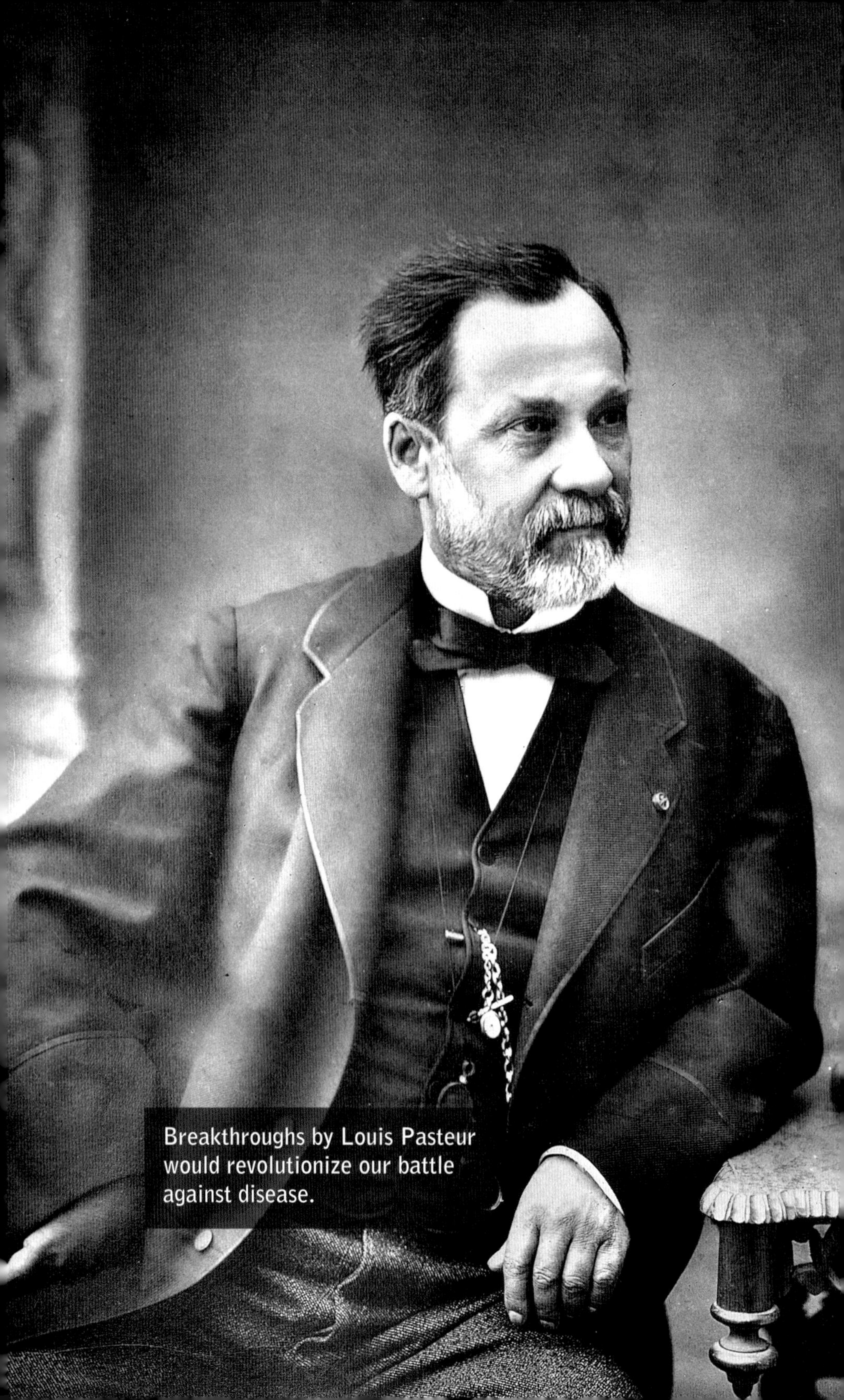

Breakthroughs by Louis Pasteur would revolutionize our battle against disease.

chemistry professor at the University of Strasbourg. In 1849, he married the daughter of the head of the university. He and Marie Laurent had five children.

Pasteur did some groundbreaking work in chemistry while at Strasbourg, and in 1854, he accepted a position as professor and dean of science at the University of Lille. It was here that he would start on the work with fermentation that eventually led him down the path to his remarkable later breakthroughs in identifying and combating disease. He continued his work when he moved to a new role as head of science back at the École Normale Supérieure where he had studied years before. It was now 1857. As it turns out, his insightful work on uncovering the role of microbes in fermentation helped save France's beer and wine industries from going broke. The emperor actually asked him to help because the producers had been unable to solve a problem with contamination that was happening.

As he continued on in his central work, making a few more shifts to different university positions, it happens that he also stepped in and helped save France's silk industry from collapse by solving a problem with disease among the silkworms. This would end up being an important stepping stone to his direct interest in infectious diseases.

ROBERT KOCH

Robert Heinrich Hermann Koch (1843–1910) was born in Germany to Mathilde Julie Henriette Biewand and Hermann Koch. He was a sharp young man and had already taught himself to write and read before he started school at the age of five. In school, he was a talented student in math and science, so he went on to study at the University of Göttingen in 1862. Though he started out majoring in science, he switched over to medicine. While studying there he had the opportunity to work with Jacob Henle, a prominent researcher on contagious disease.

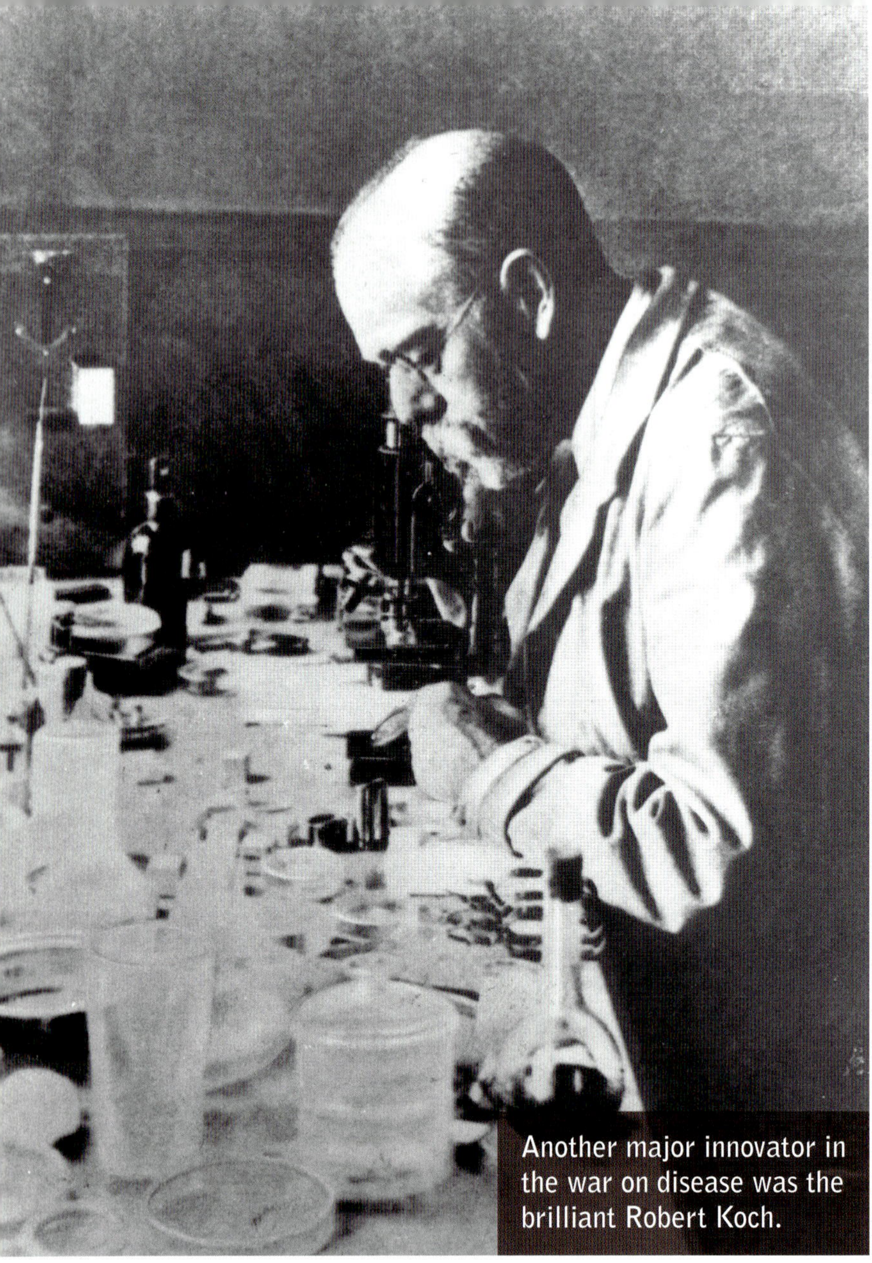
Another major innovator in the war on disease was the brilliant Robert Koch.

In 1866, Koch finished medical school, graduating with highest honors, and in 1867, he married Emma Fraatz. Their daughter, Gertrude, was born the next year. He served as a military doctor during the Franco-Prussian War (1870–1871) and then set up practice as a surgeon and built himself a small laboratory for his scientific interests. It was in this lab that his curiosity about the causes of disease would begin to develop more fully. In particular, he would begin to build on promising work by researchers like Pasteur and his old mentor Henle.

With several years of good work behind him, Koch had gained some recognition and was offered a position in the Imperial Health Office. This provided access to additional resources, including laboratory space and a strong group of colleagues. It was during his time there that he began developing ideas for guidelines that could be used to isolate the organism causing a specific disease.

In 1889, Koch met a seventeen-year-old actress named Hedwig Freiberg. He fell madly in love with Hedwig, and his wife, Emma, agreed to a divorce in 1893. Later that same year, he and Hedwig were married. She was twenty-nine years younger than Robert.

His amazing work continued, in spite of the public muttering that his divorce and remarriage had caused. In addition to his success in working to solve tuberculosis, he also took part in a German group sent to Egypt to research an outbreak of cholera. He nearly identified the specific bacterium to blame near the end of the epidemic and completed his quest in India.

After a few years of additional research and work as a professor and administrator at Berlin University, Koch died in 1910. He had pushed right to the end, though, having given a speech about his research just three days before he passed away.

WALTER REED

Walter Reed was born in 1851, in Virginia. He was the youngest of five kids. His mother was Pharaba White, and his father, Lemuel Sutton Reed, was a Methodist minister.

Walter's family moved to Charlottesville in 1866, and he started at the University of Virginia with a plan to study classics but changed over to medicine. He had a real talent for it, and he graduated in 1869. He was only seventeen—still the youngest to complete a medical degree from UVA. He then went to Bellevue Medical College in New York to build up more experience and finished his second medical degree a year later.

After considering several hospital positions, he decided on a military career and joined the Army Medical Corps in 1875 as a first lieutenant. He married Emilie Lawrence in 1876, and for the next eighteen years they hopped around to different military posts. In that time, they had a daughter and a son, and they adopted a Native American girl. Then in 1889, he was stationed in Baltimore, which gave him the opportunity to do advanced coursework on bacteria and the study of diseases.

In 1893 he became a professor at George Washington University School of Medicine, a medical school that had been set up by the army. It was during his time there that he investigated rising cases of yellow fever among the soldiers who were serving near the Potomac River. He was able to show that it was not being caused by drinking the water. Based on his strong investigation skills and this previous success, he was appointed to teams to investigate typhoid and then yellow fever. This was the work that would securely etch his name in history.

Engineers were brought in to help alleviate yellow fever in Cuba based on Reed's work, and he went back to teach in Washington, DC. He passed away after surgery on his appendix in 1902. As a testament to his contributions, the Walter Reed Hospital in Washington was named after him.

MAX THEILER

Max Theiler (1899–1972) was from Pretoria, South Africa, but actually spent most of his career living and working in the United States. He was the youngest of four children. His father was a veterinary bacteriologist and the director of South Africa's veterinary services. Both he and Max's mother, Emma Jegge, had come from Switzerland.

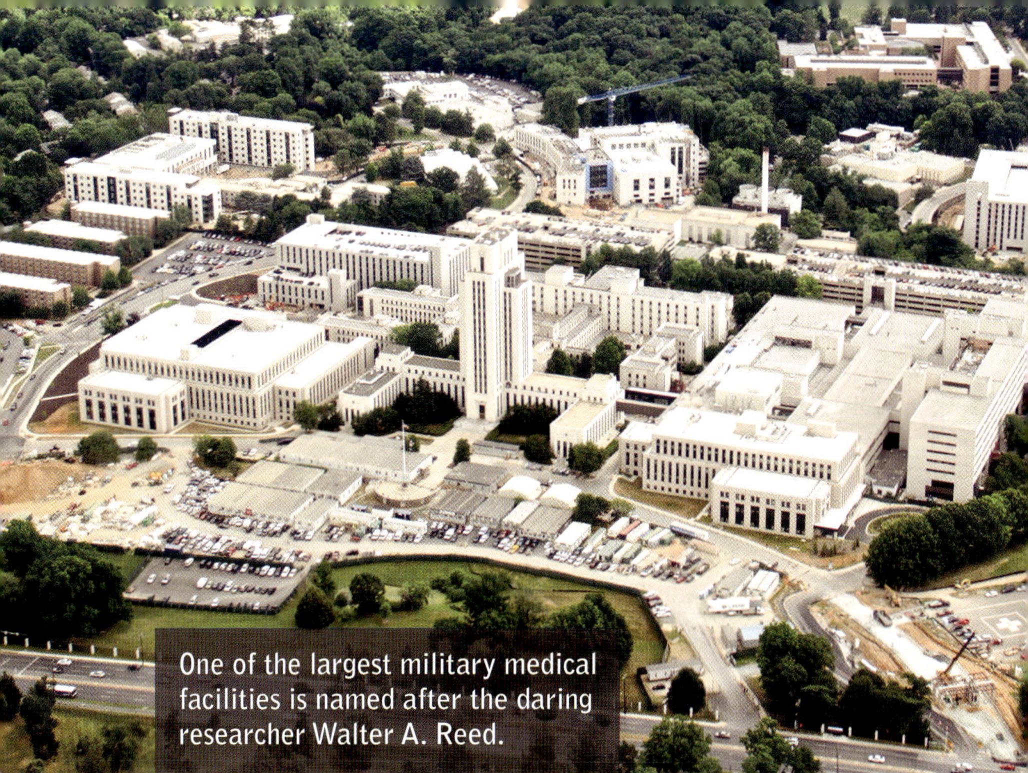

One of the largest military medical facilities is named after the daring researcher Walter A. Reed.

Largely in response to pushing from his father, Theiler attended a two-year premedical program at the University of Cape Town. He trained in medicine at St. Thomas' Hospital and at the London School of Hygiene and Tropical Medicine. When he graduated in 1922, he moved to the United States to take a position at Harvard.

It was during his time at Harvard that he did some preliminary research on yellow fever, among other things. One big breakthrough came in 1926 when he and Andrew Sellards were able to show that yellow fever was not caused by the *Leptospira icteroides* bacteria, but rather by a virus. This is also the period when he accidentally caught yellow fever (though he survived).

Theiler was hired by the Rockefeller Institute in 1930 and continued his work on yellow fever and other infectious diseases. He switched from using monkeys to mice in his experiments while he was at the Rockefeller Institute (now called Rockefeller University). This switch would have profound implications.

Theiler married Lillian Graham in 1938, and they had one daughter. He was awarded a Nobel Prize in 1951, and in 1964,

Theiler retired from the Rockefeller Foundation to become a professor at Yale, where he remained until 1967.

JONAS SALK

Jonas Edward Salk was born in 1914 in New York City. He was the eldest of three brothers. Both parents, Daniel Salk and Dora Press, were Jewish immigrants who had come over from Poland.

After attending a public school for gifted students, he earned a bachelor's degree in chemistry from City College of New York in 1934. He had skipped grades along the way, so he was only fifteen when he started college. In 1939, Salk graduated with his medical degree from New York University (the same university Walter Reed had attended). While he was studying there, he had the chance to work with Thomas Francis, whose work on using killed viruses to create immunity would play a big role in Salk's research interests.

Salk married Donna Lindsay in 1939 the day after he graduated. Lindsay was working on her master's degree in social work. They had three children together before divorcing in 1968. Salk's second wife was Françoise Gilot, a French artist and best-selling author. From 1944 to 1953, she had been Pablo Picasso's partner, and they had two children together.

In 1942, Salk became part of Thomas Francis's team at the University of Michigan. They were trying to develop a vaccine that would work against influenza, a fast-evolving viral disease responsible for several large pandemics.

Salk then took a position as an associate professor and as head of the Virus Research Laboratory at the University of Pittsburgh in 1947. The Virus Research Laboratory is where he began his research on polio, which attacked the nervous system and was impacting thousands of children every year. Among his projects was the attempt to confirm the findings of other research by identifying three distinct strains of polio. This was important because the body's immune system develops unique responses to each one.

Salk would go on to serve as a full professor of bacteriology and experimental medicine at Pittsburgh. In 1963, he took a directorship in San Diego, California, for the Institute for Biological Studies (which would later be renamed as the Salk Institute).

He was also awarded the Presidential Medal of Freedom in 1977 by then president Jimmy Carter. The other recipient that year was Martin Luther King Jr.

MAURICE HILLEMAN

Maurice Ralph Hilleman (1919–2005) was an American biologist who would be responsible for developing forty vaccines. His development of solutions to chicken pox, hepatitis A and B, measles, meningitis, **mumps**, **rubella**, and other diseases resulted in, quite literally, countless lives being saved.

Maurice was the eighth child of Gustav and Anna Hilleman, a farm family living on the plains of Montana. He had a twin sister who died at birth. He would often credit his work with chickens while growing up as the foundation for his later work using chickens in his research. His parents could not afford to send him to college, but his older brother stepped in to help make up the difference between his scholarships and the college costs. Hilleman earned his degree from Montana State University in 1941. With a fellowship to the University of Chicago, he earned his PhD in microbiology in 1944.

After graduating, he developed his first vaccine while working at the pharmaceutical company E. R. Squibb and Sons. It was for a strain of virus that was plaguing US troops in World War II. Hilleman would go on to hold positions at Walter Reed Army Medical Center (where he was the chief of respiratory diseases) and as an advisor for the World Health Organization (WHO).

While he was at Walter Reed, Hilleman's research on mutations in influenza viruses is what allowed him to realize

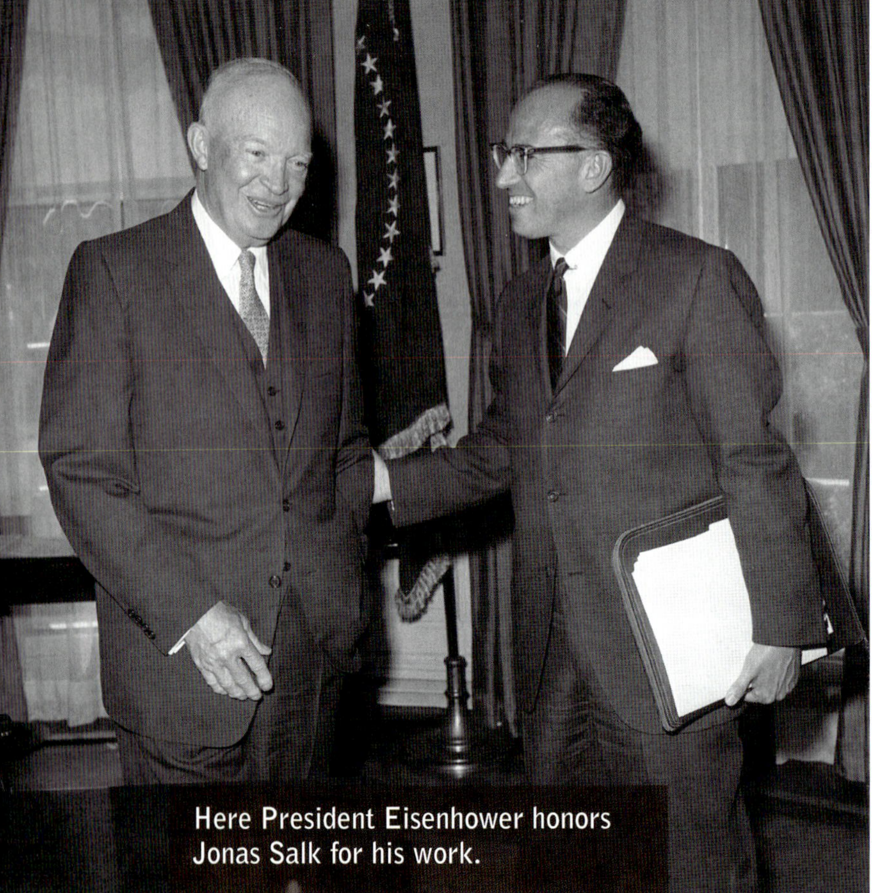
Here President Eisenhower honors Jonas Salk for his work.

sooner than other researchers how big the Hong Kong flu outbreak could be.

In 1957, he went to work for Merck and Company in New Jersey. His role as head of the virus and cell biology department provided resources and collaborators for a great many of the other vaccines he went on to create. As you might expect of someone driven enough to develop forty different vaccines, after his mandatory retirement from Merck, he spent the next twenty years as the director of the new Merck Institute for Vaccinology. When he died in 2005 at the age of eighty-five, he was also still teaching as an adjunct professor at the University of Pennsylvania.

There is a great quote from Robert Gallo, one of the two people credited with discovering the virus that causes AIDS: "If I had to name a person who has done more for the benefit of human health, with less recognition than anyone else, it would be Maurice Hilleman."

Robert Koch's Nobel Prize

In 1905, Robert Koch was awarded the Nobel Prize in Physiology or Medicine. Count K. A. H. Mörner presented Koch with the prize, giving a speech that detailed the importance of Koch's work and that work's context:

> Already before Koch had started his investigations into this disease, it had been possible to show that tuberculosis may be inoculated into animals. It was not, however, proved that it was caused by a micro-organism, and such an interpretation was contested by very distinguished investigators.
>
> Koch made his first communication concerning his research on tuberculosis in a lecture given on March 24, 1882 to the Physiological Society of Berlin. This lecture covers scarcely two pages of print, yet in it are given the proofs of the discovery of the tubercle bacillus and the description of its chief characteristics.
>
> Seldom has an investigator been able to comprehend in advance with such clear-sightedness a new, unbroken field of investigation, and seldom has someone succeeded in working on it with the brilliance and success with which Robert Koch has done this. Seldom have so many discoveries of such decisive significance to humanity stemmed from the activity of a single man, as is the case with him.

The development of injected vaccines would represent a great innovation over the process of variolation.

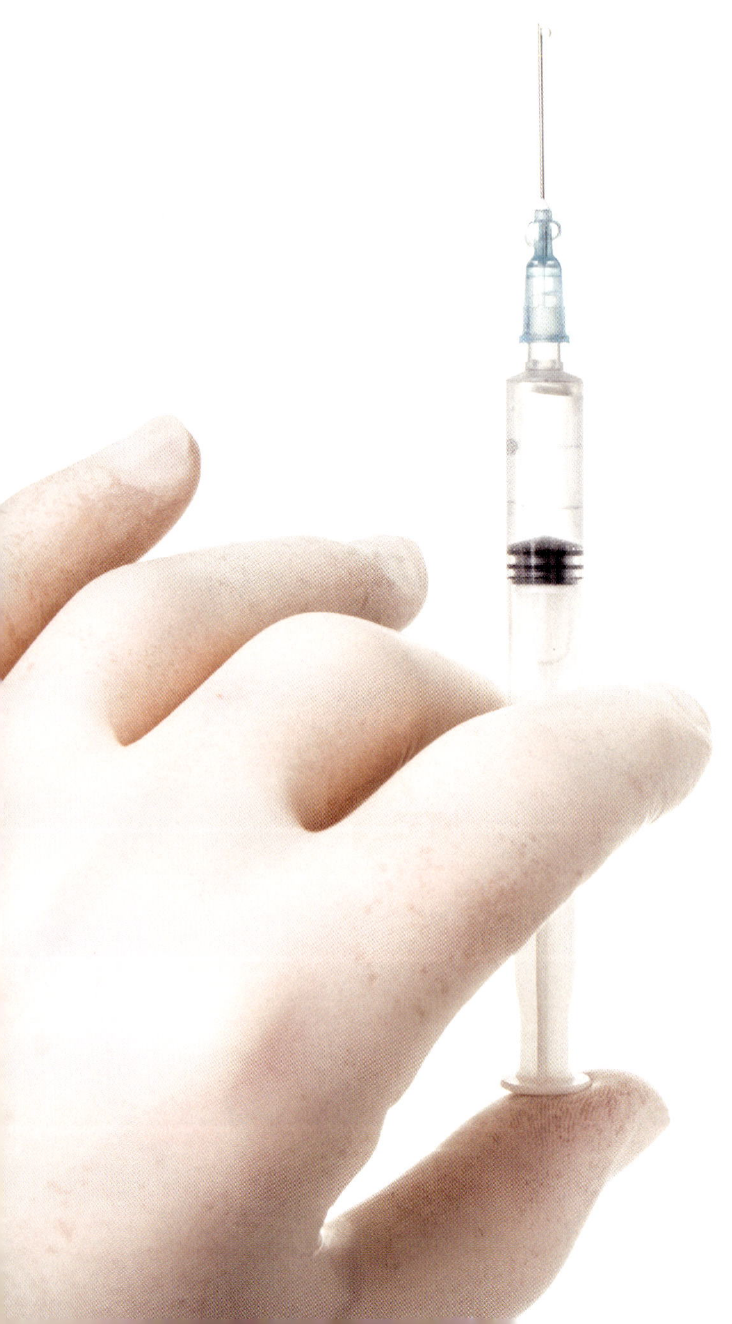

CHAPTER 4

The Discovery of Vaccines

Lady Mary Montagu was living back in England in 1718 when a smallpox epidemic was raging. You will remember that her husband was the British ambassador to Turkey and that she had been disfigured by smallpox herself years earlier and meant to save her son from the suffering and possible death. Lady Montagu first learned about variolation when they had arrived in Turkey, so she took her six-year-old son, Edward, to have the procedure done. Little did she know, she would become first in the chain of great thinkers and scientists who recognized the potential for vaccines to change the world.

LADY MONTAGU and the INFLUENCE of VARIOLATION

As we know from Lady Montagu's letters, the "procedure" (variolation) as it was practiced in Turkey was performed by a group of old women. They would scratch open a vein on the arm and then place about a pinhead worth of infected material into the opened vein. They did this for thousands of people. Lady Montagu was so thankful and so impressed by the results that she communicated with doctors back in England to try and have the practice adopted there as well.

In England, in 1721, she convinced Doctor Charles Maitland to perform the procedure on her two-year-old daughter. In spite of the powerful effects of the inoculation, Lady Montagu still suffered harsh criticism for her efforts to spread the practice. It was true that some who received the procedure still died, and, of more concern, it was possible to catch the disease from someone who had received the inoculation. There was still work to be done.

COTTON MATHER

Cotton Mather was a prominent clergyman in Boston, and he is widely credited for his role in helping to bring variolation to the new American colonies. In 1713, he wrote in his diary about his concern for the coming measles epidemic. His sense of dread was well founded, and as the disease swept through town, he lost his second wife, their infant twin daughters, another of his daughters, and the maid all within weeks of each other. This would serve as inspiration for his later efforts to combat disease.

In 1721, a smallpox epidemic erupted through Boston, taking the lives of about 850 people. Mather convinced the physician Zabdiel Boylston to use variolation to inoculate as many against the disease as he could. He had first learned about the practice from one of his slaves, back in 1706, and had then read about it in English medical journals (likely a result of Lady Montagu's efforts).

Mather's son Samuel was studying at Harvard at the time, and his chambermaid came down with smallpox. Strangely enough, Samuel's brother had to push Cotton to get Samuel inoculated. While 14 percent of the people who caught smallpox died, the rate for those who had been inoculated was only 3 percent. In spite of its positive effects, Mather's promotion of variolation aroused powerful resistance, including threatening notes and letters. On one occasion, someone threw a poorly made explosive through his front window!

To understand in context, common treatments in the late seventeenth century for smallpox included such things as draining away some of the patients' blood, making sure their covers were not pulled up higher than the waist, and giving medications that would induce vomiting or extra bowel movements. Then, of course, you have ideas like when the governor of Virginia called for a day of penance and prayer as a way to fight the measles outbreak.

In 1753, a Scottish physician named Francis Home was able to show through experimentation that measles was the result of something carried in the blood. He drew blood from an infected person and injected it under the skin of an uninfected person, who then got a mild case of the disease.

VARIOLATION among the ROYALTY

The fatality rate with variolation was often as much as a tenth that of contracting smallpox naturally; it was hardly a hard choice. Because nearly everyone was likely exposed to the disease, members of the noble families embraced variolation. Some of the royalty engaging in variolation for themselves and their children included the Empress Maria-Theresa of Austria along with her children and grandchildren, King Frederick II of Prussia (who also used it on his soldiers), and King Louis XVI of France and his children. Even Catherine II of Russia chose variolation over taking her chances with smallpox.

It was not, by any means, a perfect solution. In addition to the potential for basic infection of the wounds by which the smallpox was introduced into the body, there was also the possibility of contracting a case of smallpox stronger than victims could fight off. There were also incidents of other diseases being transmitted along with it, like syphilis.

EDWARD JENNER ADVANCES the FIELD

Edward Jenner would not exactly invent immunization, as is sometimes claimed. Rather, what he did was develop an innovation in the procedure by which it was done. Mind you, it was a tremendously valuable innovation, and it led to great breakthroughs. We should be careful, however, not to make it sound like Jenner was engaged in anything like the scientific research and analysis that we see later in figures like Koch or Reed.

At the heart of his innovation were actually two innovations. The first was to move beyond the use of things like ground scabs or crusts from wounds of people who had the disease, as had been done in places like Turkey. The second was to test out whether matter from a different, but closely related, disease could be used instead of the exact disease.

Jenner took some fluid and tissue from a cowpox sore on the hand of a local milkmaid and injected it under the skin of an eight-year-old boy named James Phipps. The boy had a reaction around the injection site, and he felt slightly ill for a few days but then recovered. At that point, Jenner then injected him with matter from a fresh human smallpox sore to see if he would come down with the illness. It was a great breakthrough for science when he did not. There was a new weapon available in our battle against disease, and for the first time an inoculation using one disease had been effective against a different one.

In 1798, the Royal Society refused to give Jenner credit for his results. Jenner, then, published a small pamphlet on his own laying out the success with Phipps and with twenty-two others. When a friend of his, another physician, **replicated** his results, word began to spread quickly.

Jenner died in 1823 at the age of seventy. As one part of his legacy, the mortality data for London shows that the number of deaths in the ten years before vaccination (1791–1800) was over eighteen thousand, but the deaths in the last measured

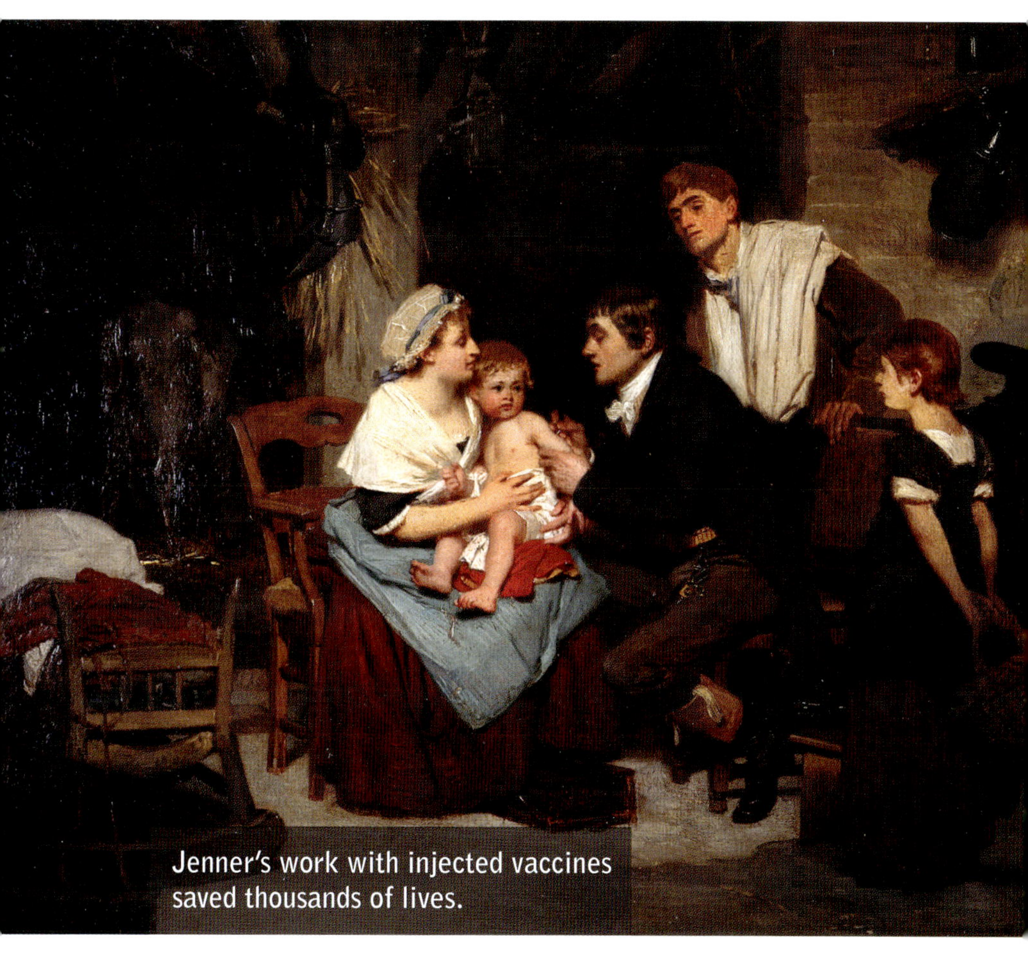

Jenner's work with injected vaccines saved thousands of lives.

decade of his life (1811–1820) were down to fewer than eight thousand. That is a 55 percent drop!

On the Heels of Jenner

In 1846, due to his work on the isolated Faroe Islands in the North Atlantic, Doctor Peter Panum was able to pin down with some accuracy the fourteen-day cycle of transmission for measles—one more small, but important victory in a long battle.

Doctor John Snow in 1849 argued for water as the transmission medium for cholera, rather than alternative theories like miasma (a cloud of contaminated air). He theorized that there were some kind of tiny particles in the water that, when ingested, were able to lodge in the body and begin multiplying.

Then, in 1854, the Italian doctor Filippo Pacini was the first to link cholera to an observable bacteria. He identified the small structures while examining the intestines of deceased cholera victims through his microscope. His characterization was of rod-like structures with a whip-like tail, or flagellum (now known by the name vibrio cholera, the *vibrio* comes from the Latin word "to quiver"). He would go on to form several true theories about the function and treatment of cholera, but his ideas were largely brushed aside at the time.

PASTEUR MAKES HIS MARK

In 1857 as the director of scientific studies at the École Normale Supérieure, Louis Pasteur's research on fermentation laid the foundation for later understanding of disease and bacteria. His first important step was to demonstrate that by heating or filtering, he could prevent the onset of fermentation or rotting. It is a tragedy and an irony that the man who would

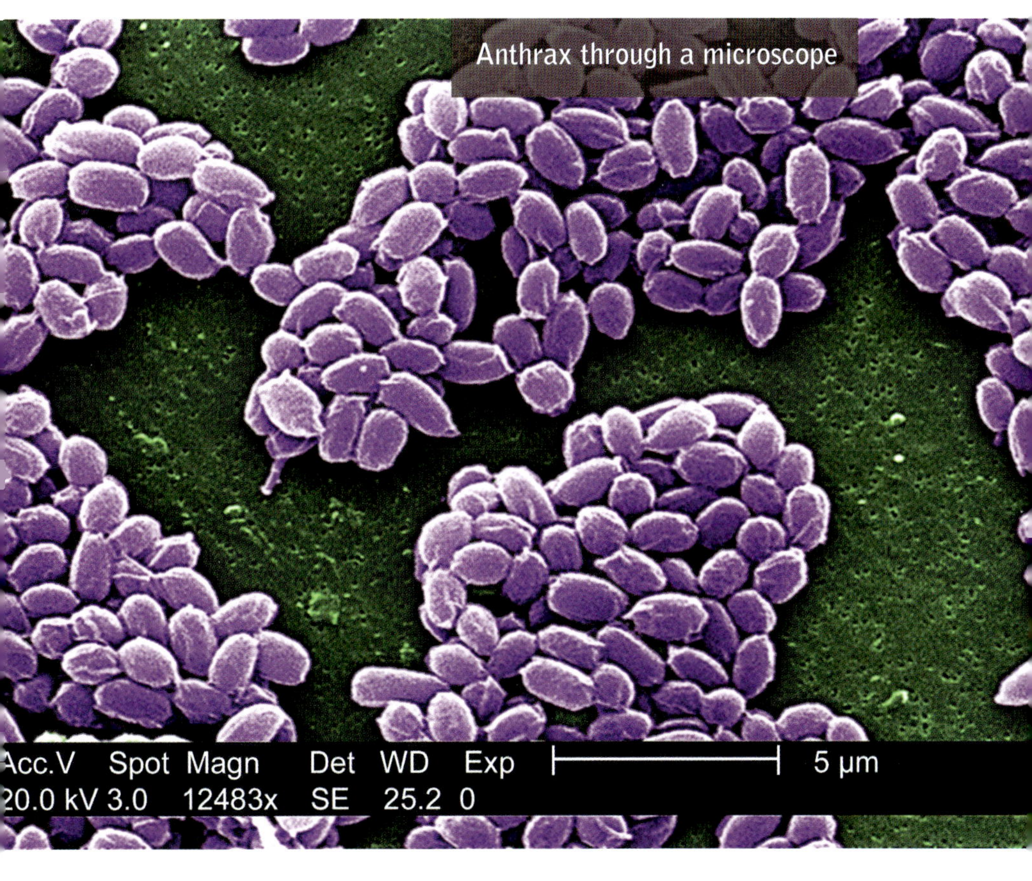

Anthrax through a microscope

do so much to help battle disease lost his own daughter to typhoid fever in 1859, when she was only nine.

It was in 1862 that Pasteur's biggest breakthrough would come. The most foundational element of his experiments was to establish that fermentation and rotting did not arise by bacteria spontaneously forming out of thin air, so to speak. That was the common theory at the time. By removing microorganisms from the samples, by heating or filtration, and then preventing microorganisms from traveling by air to reach them, he was able to show that organisms had not just formed from the air. As a result, he was awarded a prize from the French Academy of Sciences, but many scientists continued to resist his conclusions.

In 1865, Pasteur's two-year-old daughter died of a liver tumor, but then the very next year he again lost a daughter to infectious disease. This time it was twelve-year-old Cécile, who had contracted a fatal case of typhoid.

The year 1877 found Pasteur working again to defeat a ridiculous theory. Actually, there were several related theories. Many people thought anthrax, a fatal disease most common in cattle, could be caused by toxic plants, biting insects, maybe even hot weather—anything, it seems, except a microorganism. Pasteur, however, was able to corroborate work completed by Koch the previous year showing that the agent of disease was actually anthrax bacilli.

In an effort to improve on the creation and availability of vaccines, Pasteur was able to produce the first lab-sourced vaccine in 1879. In this case, it was to inoculate chickens against a particular form of cholera. This vaccine worked through the use of an attenuated (weakened) sample of the bacteria. The method of weakening was exposure to oxygen and was discovered quite by accident when a lab assistant left the bacteria out for several days before administering it.

A SERIES of TRIUMPHS

Linking Mosquitoes and Disease

In 1881, Carlos Finlay presented his research findings to the Academy of Sciences in Havana, Cuba. In his paper, he made the case that it was mosquitoes that were responsible for transmitting yellow fever. Unfortunately, his work was not taken seriously until it was corroborated by US Army researchers in the early 1900s.

Diphtheria Identified

A more significant breakthrough came in 1883, when Edwin Klebs, a Swiss-German scientist, was able to successfully identify the bacterium responsible for diphtheria. This would go hand in hand with work by Friedrich Loeffler, who was able to cultivate the diphtheria bacteria. Loeffler would go on to discover that this microorganism, now known as *Corynebacterium diphtheriae*, produces toxins that attack the cells of the host.

Homegrown Tuberculosis

In the meantime, in 1882, the brilliant researcher Robert Koch was able to isolate and identify the particular bacteria that causes tuberculosis. This bacteria now goes by the name of *Mycobacterium tuberculosae*. At the time he presented his findings, tuberculosis (often called TB for short) was killing close to one out of every seven people. Strangely, that rate was even higher among the middle-age groups.

The First Blow Against Bacteria

Jaime Ferran was the first to develop a vaccine against a bacterial disease. The others up until this point were diseases caused by viruses, like smallpox. Building on the work of

Pasteur, he managed to grow cholera bacteria in the lab and then used a series of one to three small injections to give people a mild infection. He ended up vaccinating over fifty thousand people to combat a cholera epidemic raging in Spain at the time. Ferran went on to develop vaccines for plague, rabies, **tetanus**, tuberculosis, and typhoid.

Fighting Rabies

Pasteur began the in-depth study of rabies in 1880, and by 1885 he was able to finally create a vaccine that worked on fifty different test cases on dogs without a failure.

As it happened, in July of that year, a boy of nine who had been bitten repeatedly by a rabid dog was brought in. Pasteur knew from his research, and from having seen a rabies outbreak in his youth, that the boy would not likely live. So, over the next ten days, Pasteur administered a weakened version that allowed the boy's immune system to build a response. When the boy lived, Pasteur was hailed as a hero and he went on to conduct more human trials.

In 1886, he was able to show the results. His vaccination had been tested on 350 people with only one fatality. That death, he believed, was the result of the person receiving the vaccine too late to prevent the disease. Rabies had been rather difficult, since there is substantial variation in the length of time between being infected and the onset of symptoms. In order to reach that point in his research, he first had to work to cultivate samples of the strongest strains of rabies so the timeline for running the tests would be easier to control during his experiments.

Healed with Poison

A two-man team in 1883, Émile Roux and Alexandre Yersin, discovered that the toxins given off by diphtheria could cause some of the symptoms of diphtheria—the membrane that forms blocking the throat, the internal bleeding, and others—when administered to animals.

In 1890, another two-man research team, Shibasaburo Kitasato and Emil von Behring, was able to develop a vaccine using just the toxin from diphtheria after heating it to make it weaker. Their work was the first time this type of solution had been developed. Their second breakthrough was more amazing because they went on to show that injecting an animal with the **serum** from an immunized animal would also provide immunity. Their third, and most significant, breakthrough, though, was to show that injecting an infected animal with blood from one that had immunity could cure the disease.

More Work with Mosquitoes

In 1900, Walter Reed and the US Army Yellow Fever Commission were tasked with solving the puzzle of yellow fever. The incredibly high death toll during the Spanish-American War was the inspiration for the army to get involved. The group visited with Carlos Finlay, who had posited mosquitoes as the disease carrier. This was tricky because at first the mosquitoes who had fed on infected hosts did not seem to pass on the disease when they then fed on a healthy person. As it turned out, however, the mosquitoes could not pass on the disease until at least twelve days after taking it in. That minimum varied, though, and sometimes the disease would not be passed on until as long as twenty days after the mosquito had fed on an infected person.

Not only were Reed and his team able to test out and confirm Finlay's theory, but they also went on to conduct studies that ruled out the possibility that it was a bacteria that was at the root of the disease. This was, as a result, the first human virus identified. The mosquito control programs that were then implemented to help control the disease also caused a drop in malaria. Those same programs would be vital to the completion of the Panama Canal in 1904. The French had turned the project over to the United States five years earlier because of the excessive number of deaths from yellow fever and malaria.

At Long Last, Vaccines for Polio and Yellow Fever

In 1908, it would be two Viennese scientists—Karl Landsteiner and Erwin Popper—who were able to determine that polio was also caused by a virus. They took the spinal fluid from a patient who had died from polio, and in a manner familiar from other cases, they ran it through filters that were known to trap any bacteria. Yet, when they injected the filtered spinal fluid into laboratory monkeys, the monkeys came down with polio. Their theory could not be confirmed until the 1950s when electron microscopes made it possible to see viruses.

It was not until 1921 that the first human tests of a vaccination against tuberculosis were ready; Albert Calmette and Camile Guérin had developed an attenuated form of the bacteria that causes TB in cows.

Around the same time, Max Theiler had to make two breakthroughs in order to come up with a vaccine against yellow fever. The first, in 1930, was to prove that yellow fever could be given to lab mice. Up until then, researchers had been using monkeys, which were much more expensive and much more difficult to handle. The second, in 1936, was to eventually develop an attenuated virus from chicken embryos. This was, of course, one of the many strains that he was able to test on lab mice first. After the results of his human trials were published in 1937, his vaccine became the standard one.

Preliminary trials for the polio vaccine were completed by 1954, and it was rolled out to large-scale testing. Just over

1.25 million school children were put into groups for a test of Salk's polio vaccine. One group got the vaccine, one got a placebo, and a smaller control group got no shot at all. Students who received a shot did not know whether it was real or placebo, nor did the teachers, the parents, or the health officials administering the vaccinations. It would take a year before the results could be analyzed and the vaccine declared 80 percent to 90 percent effective against polio.

WHAT IS HAPPENING INSIDE?

Now that we have a sense of the unfolding development of different breakthroughs that allowed science to identify the pathogens of these diseases and develop solutions to fight them, let us walk through a basic discussion of why and how these solutions—these vaccines—actually work.

While "vaccines" and "vaccination" were named by Jenner based on the cowpox virus he worked with (*Variolae vaccinae*), Pasteur thought the terms should be used to refer to *all* inoculations against contagious disease—Pasteur's ground-breaking rabies vaccine included.

Let us get a clearer handle on what we mean when we use these terms because they sometimes get stretched to mean the same thing as "immunization." Immunization is a larger category. It includes both the development of immunity as a result of getting an injection to provoke the body's response mechanisms and the development of such response mechanisms due to natural infection.

"Vaccine," then, refers to a biological substance that develops acquired immunity to a particular disease. In particular, it develops an active immunity. That means the actual defense mechanisms are produced by the patient's own system. Vaccines can contain one of several kinds of ingredient that will achieve this. A vaccine can contain a weakened or dead form of the pathogen. It can contain small amounts of the toxins that are produced by the pathogen. Or, it can contain some of the proteins from the pathogen. The last thing would be to allow that it doesn't have to be the exact pathogen itself. As was the case with Jenner's cowpox, the triggering ingredient could be from a closely related pathogen.

Once in the body these components, called **antigens**, cause the patient's own immune system to shift into gear and mobilize different possible defensive measures. Once the disease has been blocked, the patient's body retains the ability to more quickly recognize and defeat that same disease next time.

The defensive measures we are concerned with here can be broken down into three kinds of specialized cells:

- Macrophages
- B-lymphocytes, called B-cells
- T-lymphocytes, called T-cells

Macrophages swallow the virus, for example, and they can be seen on the cell surface. This causes the system to activate helper T-cells. Next in line comes the activation of B-cells and T-cells. The antibodies are then made by plasma cells that derive from the B-cells. The body keeps a few million (or a billion) of these antibodies in memory as a way of being prepared for future invasions. So the system has all these B-lymphocytes circulating at a given time. Each has a unique antibody that it carries on the surface. Whenever one bumps into the antigen it was designed to defend against, the B-cell divides into plasma cells, and each plasma cell starts producing huge numbers of antibodies to do the fighting.

This little navy of antibodies travels around the body looking for any invaders in the blood or in the spaces between cells. When they find one, a group of them latches onto the surface of the microbe so it is unable to unlock the door to invade any host cells. The antibodies also send out a signal for macrophages to come kill and eat the invader.

A Game of Hide and Seek

Cases where the invader has already gotten into host cells have to be handled by T-lymphocytes. Since these T-cells were "programmed" by being exposed to the antigen, they can detect when the body's cells have microbes inside. These microbes unlocked the cell door and snuck in to use the cell's resources for making more microbes.

Each microbe has its own individual antigens, like a chemical fingerprint. That is why vaccines have to be developed separately for each one. Once the macrophage consumes almost all the parts of the microbe, it stores the antigens. The macrophage then transports the antigens back to a lymph node and spits them out. This makes it possible for the other specialized white blood cells (B-cells and T-cells) to recognize them.

When a patient has developed immunity by responding to a vaccination or to an actual infection, the body keeps some of the T-cells. These cells, called "memory cells" are a head start for the next time the body encounters the same microbe.

Kinds of Vaccines

Coming out of the amazing stretch of science since Jenner's first solution, vaccines are one of five main types:

- Live, weakened vaccines: referred to as attenuated. These are samples of living viruses that are treated

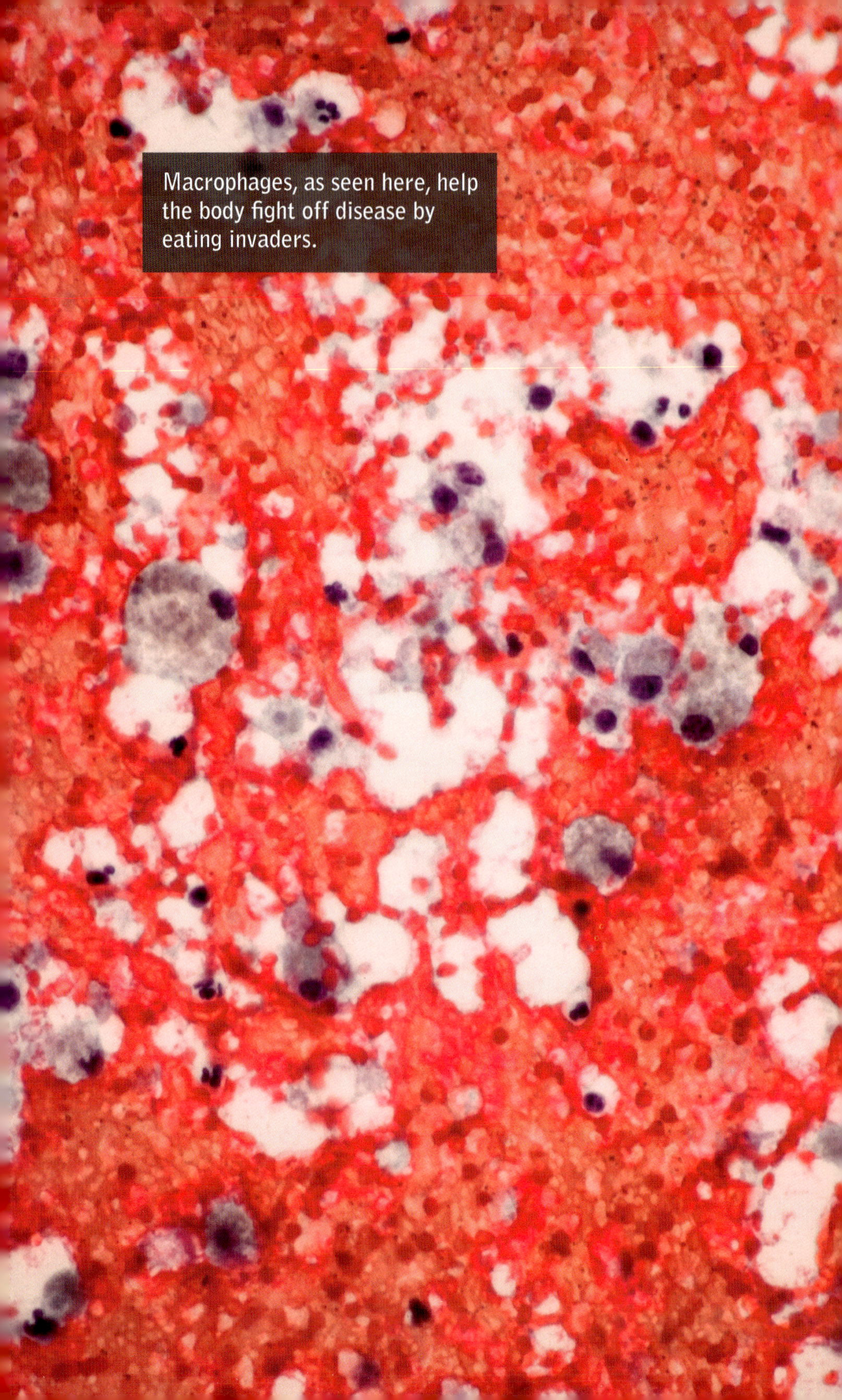

Macrophages, as seen here, help the body fight off disease by eating invaders.

in different ways to weaken their ability. Vaccines that fall into this group include chickenpox and the combined vaccine for measles, mumps, and rubella.

- Inactivated vaccines: these have been killed, but they are still capable of triggering a response. These are somewhat safer than attenuated vaccines, but there are many cases where they did not work for a given disease. Examples where inactivated vaccines do work include pertussis and some strains of influenza.

- Toxoid vaccines: These are the ones that do not even use the actual bacteria. They take the toxins (poisons) produced by the pathogen and alter it to become harmless. Vaccines that work using this strategy are given for tetanus and diphtheria.

- Subunit vaccines: For diseases like hepatitis B and human papilloma virus (HPV), the vaccine uses only part of the virus to trigger the body's response system.

- Conjugate vaccines: In these cases the scientists are able to attach a molecule to an inactivated microbe (the process is called conjugation, which just means "joining together"). The extra molecule attachment stimulates an increased immune response. These are used in cases like pneumococcus and meningococcus.

For most of these, it usually takes several doses to build up a sufficient defense. In the case of pertussis and tetanus, among others, the defense wears down over time, so they need an additional dose—a booster.

Because the vaccination is triggering the body's immune system, sometimes the side effects include normal immune responses like a low-grade fever and swelling or tenderness at the site of the inoculation. At the same time, protection is not instantaneous, so it is possible that someone who was naturally infected before the response has been established could still get the full version of the disease. (Remember the situation with Pasteur's rabies vaccination group?)

In the early 1900s, children in the United States and other Western nations would have gotten just one vaccine, smallpox, which contained about two hundred different antigens. Nowadays, smallpox vaccine is no longer given, but by the time they are teenagers, today's kids will have gotten fourteen different vaccines. These vaccines still come up to fewer antigens (160) than the old smallpox shot. While that might sound like a lot, some context will help. A child will encounter thousands and thousands of antigens from his or her normal environment.

We have around one thousand different species of bacteria, which translates to one hundred billion bacteria living on our surface and inside of us. That means we support almost one hundred times more bacteria than there are cells in our whole body. Estimates are that a healthy human body could potentially manufacture about ten billion different antibodies, and over the course of our lives we normally only produce between one million and one hundred million. There is a lot of unused capability!

PROTECTED by the HERD

There is another interesting dynamic that factors into the way vaccines help to protect us from various epidemic diseases, and that is something known as herd immunity. The idea behind this is that an occasional person who has not been immunized against a particular disease is still sheltered, in a way, when a certain percentage of the group overall *has* been immunized. For example, if around 70 percent or more of a population is vaccinated against polio, then the chance of ever coming into contact with it is very

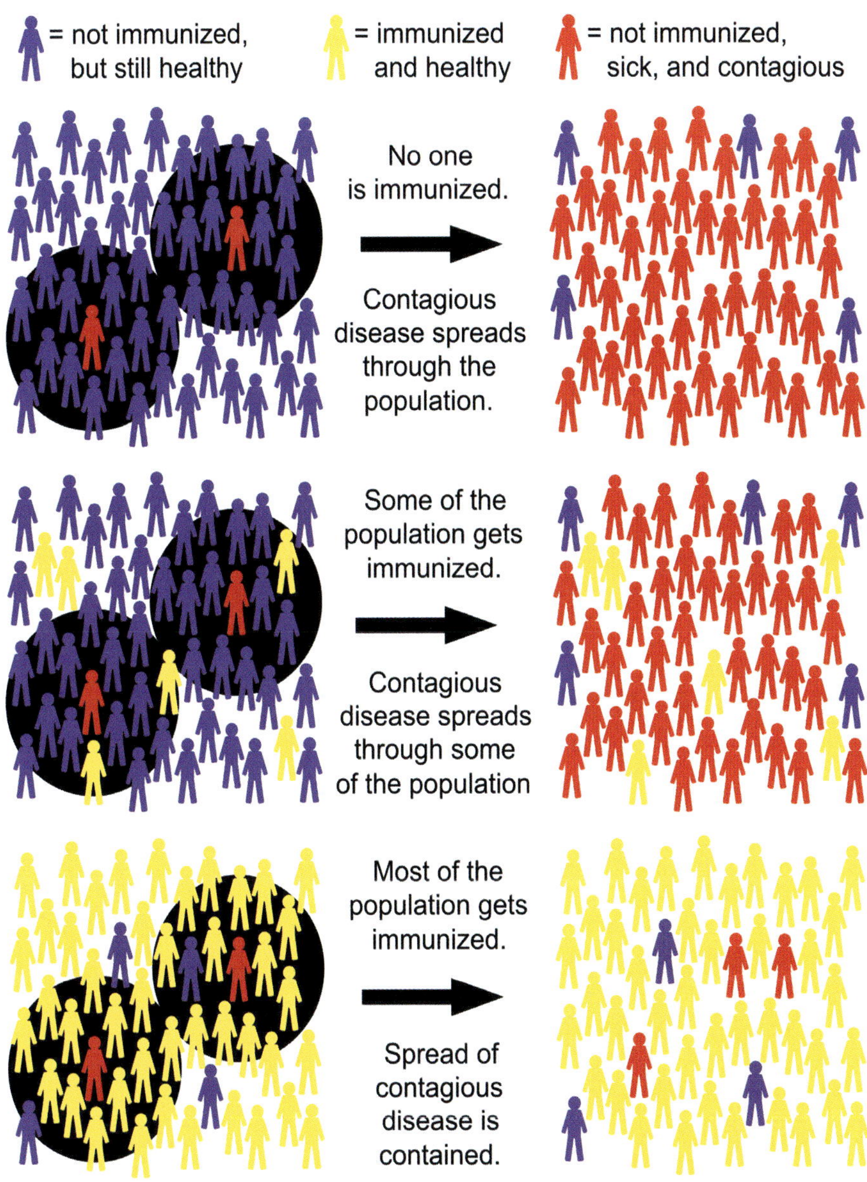

Because some people are not capable of undergoing vaccination, they depend on the shield created by others who are able to.

low. This percentage is different for each disease, though, and is referred to as the herd immunity threshold (HIT).

Herd immunity does not soften the need for every person who can to get vaccinated. Rather, it creates a buffer to help protect individuals in the group who are not able to get their shots for certain diseases—maybe they are too young or maybe their immune system is too weakened due of other illness. Key examples of this include pertussis. Infants are too young to receive the vaccine yet, but making sure programs inoculate adults above a certain percentage reduces the infants' likelihood of getting it. Another problem arises with flu vaccines, not because old people and young people are too weak to receive the vaccination, but because their immune systems are too weak to build an adequate response even if they do.

The concept was first developed in the 1920s and 1930s, partly in response to a sudden drop in new cases of measles as the percentage of people being vaccinated went up. As a result of this discovery and research that followed, herd immunity is now an intentional part of vaccination programs and policies. It is part of the justification behind having vaccination requirements for school attendance, among other things.

HEADING toward TODAY and TOMORROW

In the next chapter, we will turn to look at some of the continuing topics and obstacles in the ongoing arms race to develop vaccine weapons faster than viruses and viewpoints can adapt to block them.

As with the discussion of which scientists to consider, so, too in this chapter and the next, there were far too many victories—both small and large—to include. In considering what the key takeaways from chapter four are, perhaps it would be this last one, about herd immunity, because it pushes us to realize that medical decisions and behaviors have consequences beyond our own bodies. Just like in actual war, victory (or defeat) is a team effort. Probably before reading this chapter, you had never thought about how getting a flu shot, for instance, could save someone's baby from dying. You might not even have thought about the fact that some people aren't able to get shots for themselves.

The Electron Microscope

Although researchers had detected the presence and effect of viruses much earlier, they could not be seen until 1939. In 1931, Ernst Ruska built the first electron microscope (EM) with his advisor, Max Knoll. It would be eight years, though, before Ruska and two of his colleagues were able to actually make out the image of a virus (tobacco mosaic virus). This opened the door to many other future discoveries, such as seeing the difference between the smallpox virus and the chickenpox virus (1948) and the first image of the polio virus (1952).

An electron microscope works similarly to a regular light-based microscope. Instead of shining light through a thin specimen, though, we beam electrons through it (hence the name). Since electrons are tinier than photons the effect is like switching from 100 pixels per square inch to 1,000 pixels per square inch—way more resolution!

Because of the differences, the electron microscope has to be different in three other ways. The first is that since we can't actually register electrons with the human eye the way we can see light waves, there is a special plate that registers the electrons hitting against it. Second, the electron beam needs to be focused onto a small area of the specimen. Instead of using reflective mirrors like we would with light, we have to use magnets. Then the third major difference is because electrons can be easily deflected by air, the process of beaming and receiving them all has to happen inside a vacuum.

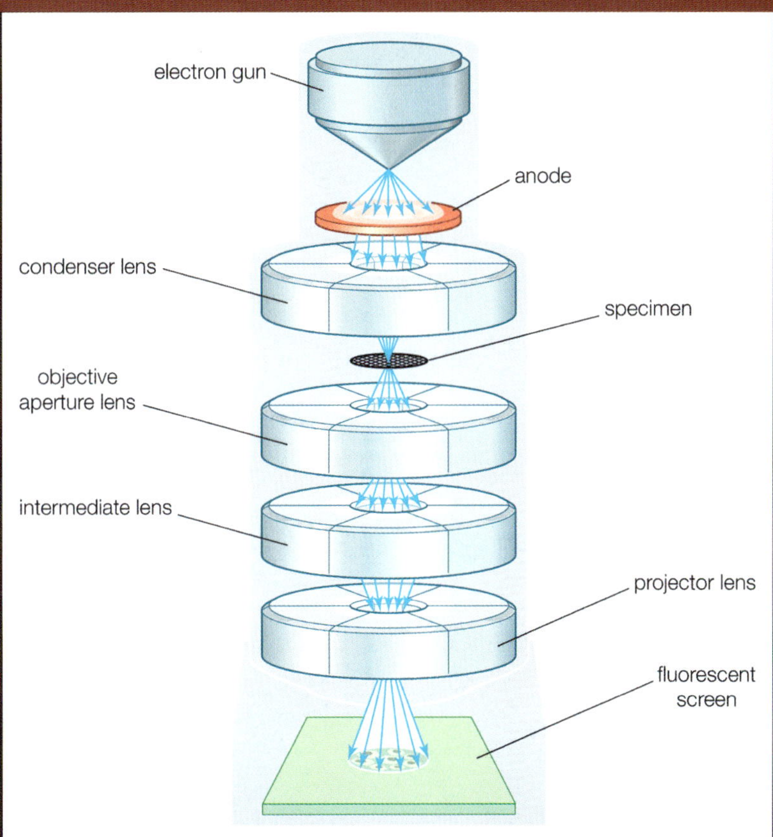

It was not until the amazing electron microscope that scientists could finally see the viruses that evidence had told them were present.

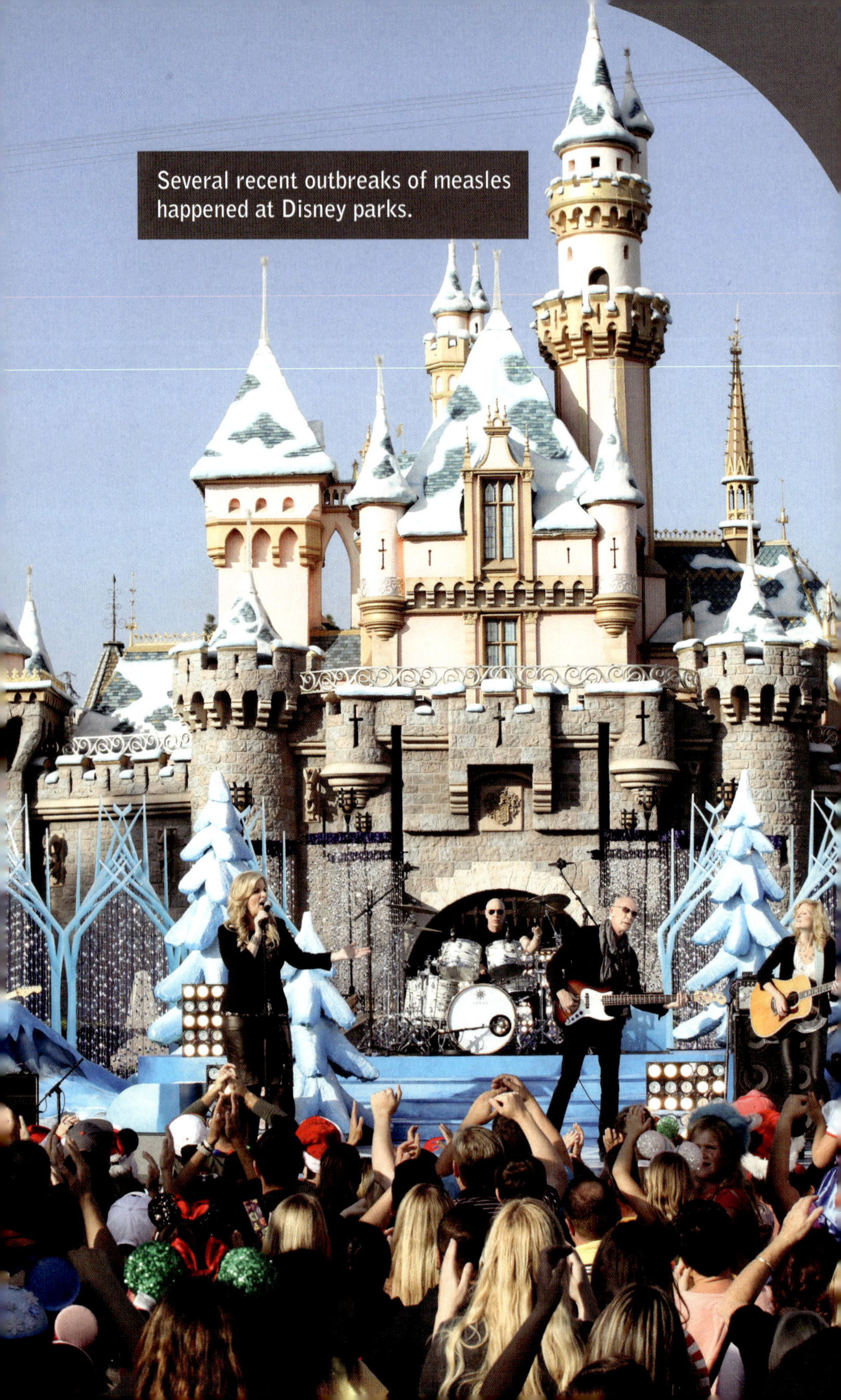

Several recent outbreaks of measles happened at Disney parks.

CHAPTER 5

The Influence of Vaccination Today

Here in the last chapter, we will look at a couple of big victories as well as get some sense of where the largest current dangers lie. Keep in mind the kinds of problems discussed at the beginning of the book about new diseases emerging and population conditions growing worse. Because of those factors, it is important to build better vaccines for existing diseases in order to stay ahead of them. It is also important to improve strategies for tackling new ones.

MAJOR DEVELOPMENTS in the POST-SALK ERA

The Asian flu pandemic struck in 1957. While this was not the first worldwide flu epidemic, it was important because Maurice Hilleman and his team determined that this was a new mutation of the influenza virus and that most people had never developed antibodies to combat it. The only people who seemed to have any resistance were a few elderly people who had been alive during the 1889 flu pandemic. Hilleman quickly sent samples of the virus to drug companies with data showing how short the window for vaccine development was (he estimated four months).

As the epidemic spread over the next two years, there were more than two million deaths, including around seventy thousand in the United States. Without Hilleman's efforts, it would have been much worse. The death toll in the United States, for example, would have reached a million or more.

Measles-Mumps-Rubella Vaccine

In 1958, the first measles vaccine was developed and tested. Doctor Sam Katz and his team in Boston ran their test on a group of eleven children. All eleven did develop the necessary antibodies, but they also developed some of the symptoms of measles. That pointed out to the researchers the need to weaken the vaccine more. More effective vaccines would be developed by John Enders and Maurice Hilleman in 1962 and 1963. The success with measles was followed closely by Hilleman's development of a mumps vaccine in 1966.

Rubella is a disease we have not discussed yet, but there was a large outbreak between 1962 and 1965 in the United States. It is normally not a particularly dangerous disease for adults, but if a woman catches rubella while pregnant it can have horrible effects. During the outbreak, more than twenty thousand children were born with a whole range of health issues, including autism, congenital heart disease, cognitive disability, deafness, eye problems, and several others. More than ten thousand women had miscarriages or chose to have abortions because of the damage and suffering the disease would cause for their babies.

By 1969, Hilleman and his research team had developed a vaccine that was in public use, and in 1971, the MMR

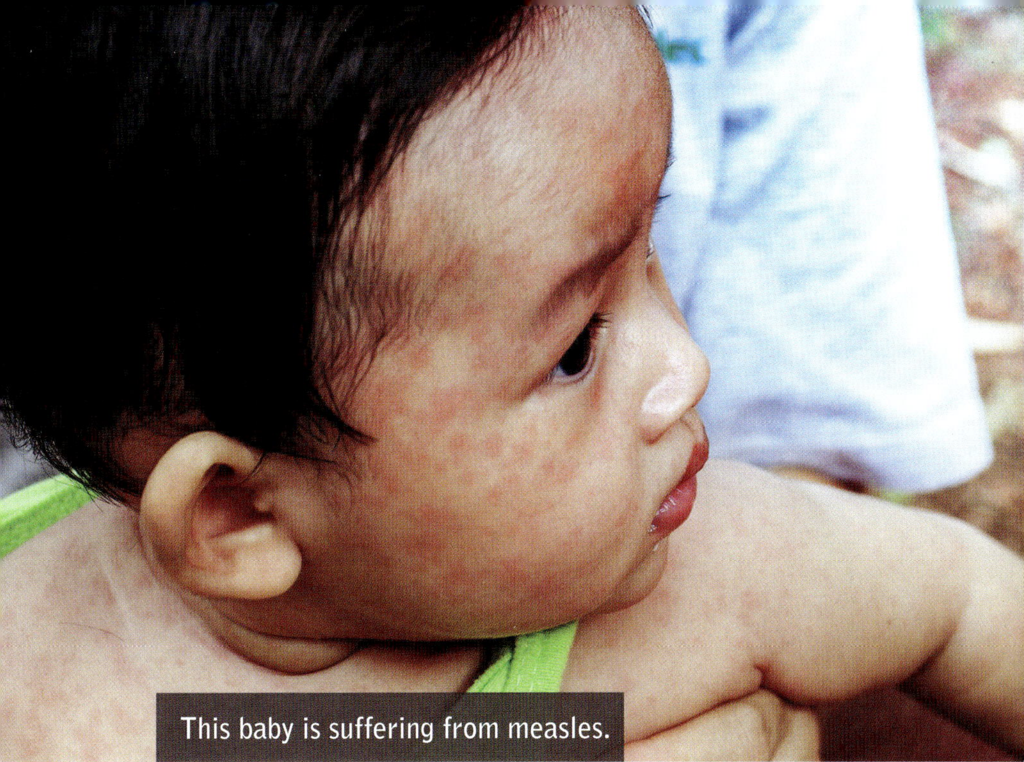

This baby is suffering from measles.

vaccination was developed to provide coverage for measles, mumps, and rubella all in one shot.

HIV: A New Front in the War

HIV and AIDS exploded into public awareness in the 1980s. The first few cases of a rare lung infection appeared in Los Angeles, California. This was part of a trail that would uncover further evidence of a breakdown in people's immune systems. By 1984, the total number of AIDS cases had reached almost eight thousand and just a little over three thousand five hundred deaths in the United States. In 1989, the total had climbed to almost four hundred thousand cases around the world and the number of reported cases in the United States hit one hundred thousand.

Since 1981, there have been over twenty-five million deaths from AIDS, putting this on the scale of the historic pandemics discussed at the beginning of the book. In 2002, AIDS was ranked as having the highest death toll for infectious diseases in Africa. While the number of new cases per year has certainly declined since the initial explosion, there were still more than thirty-nine thousand people diagnosed with HIV in the United States in 2015 (that is down from around fifty thousand in 2005).

The human immunodeficiency virus (HIV) works by actually invading and destroying the T-lymphocytes (T-cells) that are meant to help fight off invaders. This would be the equivalent of setting fire to the fire station. Like other viruses, it invades these cells and switches them over to make more copies of the virus. They then move out and invade other immune cells, and so on. Not only does that prevent the immune system from being able to effectively fight off the HIV, but it prevents it from being able to fight off any other invaders as well. That is where AIDS comes in because people who have HIV don't usually die from it directly—they die from any number of other diseases they come in contact with, like the rare lung infection mentioned.

Based on research at the Pasteur Institute and others, the US secretary of Health and Human Services declared in 1984 that there would be a vaccine available within two years. Unfortunately, the scientists working on the project ran into a number of problems that prevented that. Perhaps the most straightforward obstacle is that killed HIV does not work to provoke a sufficient immune response. The traditional alternative in that case is to use a weakened version, but so far there have been no attenuated versions that are deemed safe enough to administer widely.

While some vaccines have been developed and tested, they have run into three major features of HIV that make it particularly difficult to create a sufficient solution. One problem is that the virus is able to mutate quickly. It reproduces lightning fast, and it is a little sloppy about it, so it accumulates

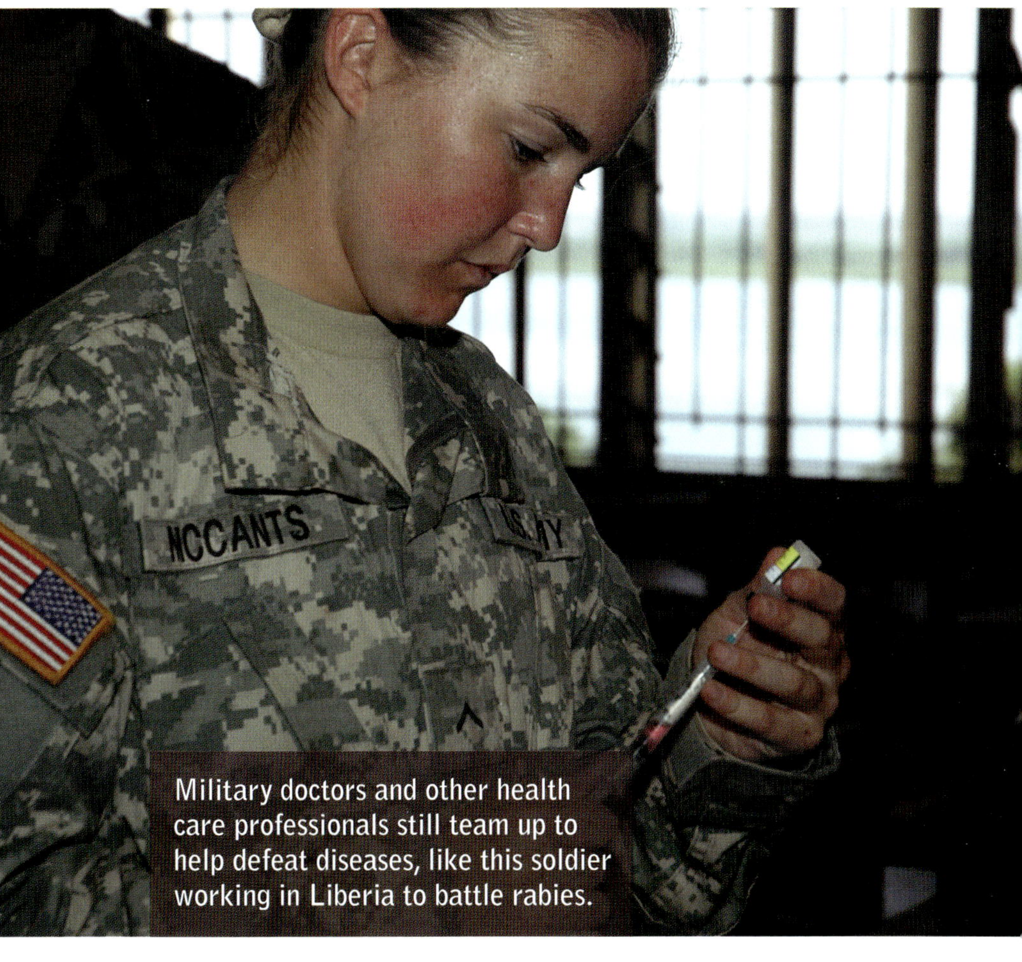

Military doctors and other health care professionals still team up to help defeat diseases, like this soldier working in Liberia to battle rabies.

lots of tiny mutations as it goes. In addition to this, it also covers itself in a kind of coating or envelope that is constantly changing. With those two advantages, that means it is changing too fast for the antibodies and the T-cells to keep up with it. The third problem is that there is a wide genetic variety within the virus, so a vaccine would have to trigger the production of immunity to a large number of particular versions.

Researchers have reason to believe that a vaccine could be effective in combating HIV. Some experiments using monoclonal antibodies provide evidence that the human body is capable of mounting a defense. This is supported by the number of people who test positive for HIV but go years and even decades without ever developing symptoms.

STATUS of BATTLES AGAINST OTHER MAJOR DISEASES

Smallpox

By combining widespread vaccination programs with practices like quarantine, smallpox had been erased from most of Europe and the United States by the 1950s. The last documented case in America was in 1949, and in 1972, the United States stopped routinely vaccinating children.

Since the specific virus affects only humans, with no place it can live in the environment or in animals, we had an advantage over it. In the 1960s, there was awareness and optimism that we might be able to wipe out smallpox altogether. The World Health Organization spearheaded a global campaign starting in 1967. After twelve years, the WHO announced that smallpox had been eradicated and recommended the end of vaccinations.

Rabies

While there are still thousands of deaths each year from rabies, nearly all of them are in countries with limited access to health care. The impact of rabies vaccines in the United States, by contrast, has been amazing. Before 1960, most cases of rabies were in domestic animals (pets), but now, around 90 percent of all cases are found only in wildlife. Because of the widespread use of vaccination after being exposed, the number of human deaths has fallen from over one hundred per year in the early 1900s to three or fewer.

Yellow Fever

Yellow fever has been stamped out everywhere except a few tropical regions in Africa and South America. In those locations, it is able to remain in certain populations of mosquitoes and monkeys. Overall there are an estimated thirty thousand deaths every year—nearly all of them are people living in those areas of South America and Africa. Since there is no treatment for yellow fever, efforts are focused on prevention—not just by vaccination, but also through steps like suppressing the mosquito population with screens on windows and doors.

Because there can be serious side effects from the vaccine, and because the chances of exposure are so low, people are usually only vaccinated if they are headed toward those tropical areas.

Typhoid

A much bigger culprit on the fatality list is typhoid. This disease currently breaks out in a little over twenty million people a year, and of those about 10 percent die. It is very uncommon in the United States, though. The number of annual cases in the United States is around three hundred every year—almost all of them from traveling.

Cholera

There are between one million and four million cases of cholera each year, and of those the deaths bounce around between twenty-eight thousand and one hundred and forty thousand per year. While there was a vaccine developed in the nineteenth century, it has only a short duration of effectiveness.

Diphtheria

In 1921, there were over two hundred thousand cases of diphtheria in the United States alone, with over fifteen thousand deaths that year. Most of those were children. Not only is that a large number, but it represents an even higher percentage of the population than it would now. In contrast, the last few decades have seen an average of less than five cases per year.

Sadly, the disease still plays a slightly larger role around the world. In 2011, for instance, the World Health Organization had reports of almost five thousand cases. When we gauge for the additional cases that probably went unreported, the number is even higher. The percentage of victims that die from the disease has held rather steady over the past forty years or so, and that ranges between 5 and 10 percent. If we look at the weaker groups, like children under five or adults past the age of forty, the fatality rate goes up closer to 20 percent.

Pertussis

Overall, pertussis has one of the more cheerful outcomes. Between 1940 and 1945, pertussis cases in the United States topped one million. With the use of vaccines, the average had fallen from around two hunded thousand per year to just a bit over one thousand in 1976.

The rates have begun climbing back up, though, in the lingering aftermath of a scare that was generated by half-baked research. This helped fuel antivaccination attitudes, and there were so many lawsuits being leveled that companies were dropping out of the pertussis vaccination market. The research was shown to be faulty, and government action limited the lawsuit maximums, which allowed some pharmaceutical companies to remain or return to the marketplace. By the year 2012, the number of cases in the United States had climbed back up to just over forty-eight thousand. This includes a large percentage of children who have not been vaccinated or have not had all their vaccinations. As we will see later in this chapter, this is part of a larger, ongoing battle.

Polio

Encouraged by the success of various vaccination programs, international health organizations launched a focused effort in 1988 to eradicate polio as had been done with smallpox. While the annual number of cases of polio in the United States had been as high as fifty-eight thousand in the 1950s, the last reported case was in 1993.

These efforts have been slowed down by ongoing wars in different regions like Pakistan and Afghanistan because these conflicts lead to the spread of disease. The efforts at eradication have also been harmed by the spread of rumors that vaccination against polio can lead to HIV or to sterilization. Currently two of the three types of polio virus appear to have been wiped out.

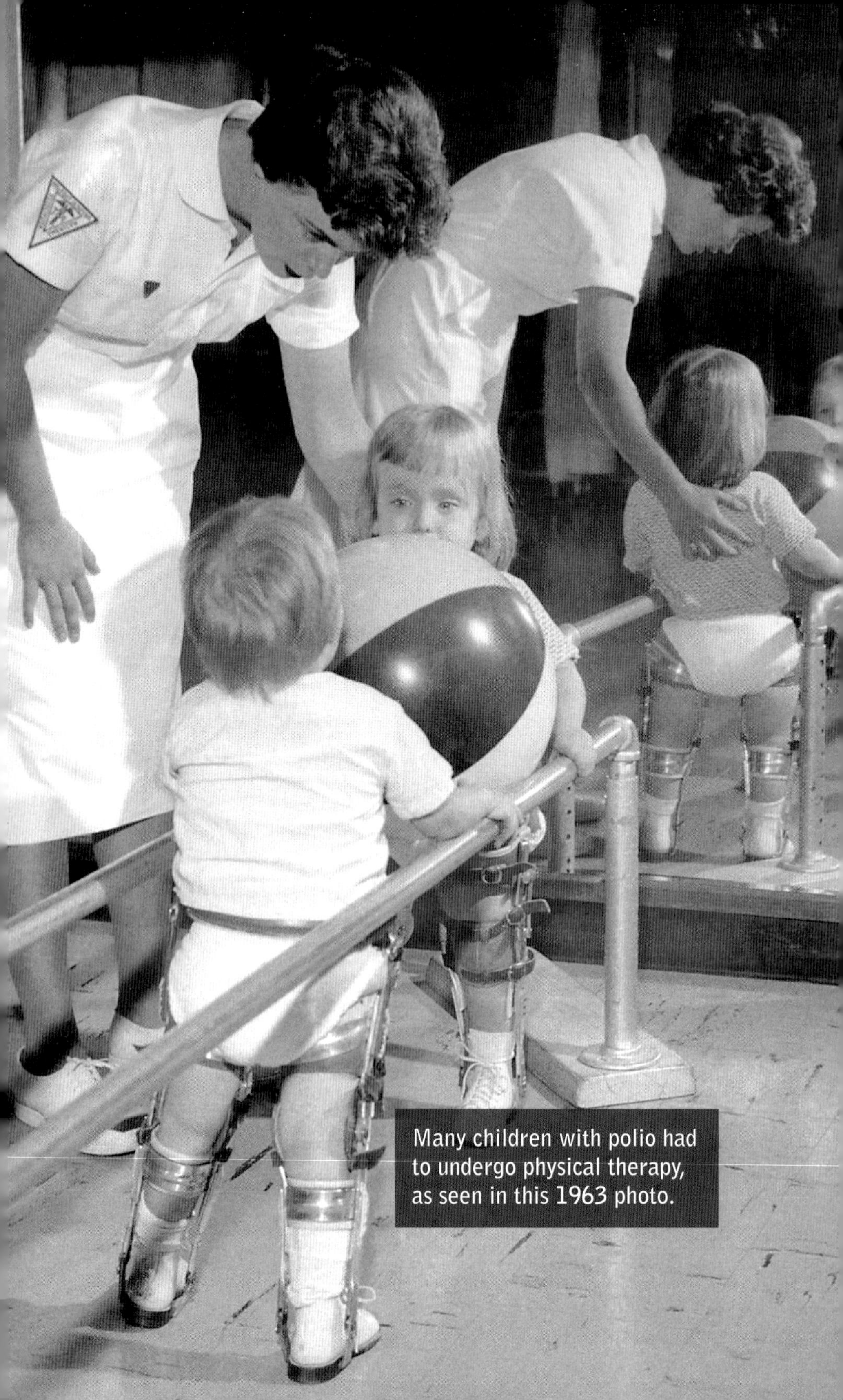

Many children with polio had to undergo physical therapy, as seen in this 1963 photo.

Measles

While the death rate from measles is around two per one thousand cases, it has harmful side effects that make it more dangerous. Pneumonia as a complication of measles took the lives of as many as one out of twenty young children with the disease. In 1958 there were over seven hundred thousand cases of measles, but once the vaccine was introduced in 1963, that number began dropping. There were only thirty-seven cases in the United States in 2004.

Worldwide deaths from measles (and complications) fell 75 percent from 2000 to 2013. They went from a little over five hundred thousand to less than one hundred and fifty thousand. Though that is the number of deaths, there are still around twenty million people who get measles every year.

The ONGOING BATTLE against UNREASON

The struggle in courts and the public sentiment against vaccination programs goes back almost to the beginning. In the United States, one of the first big legal cases came up in 1809, and they have been going ever since!

Massachusetts implemented the first law requiring immunization in the United States. This made it a legal obligation for everyone to receive a smallpox vaccination. Close on its heels, other states soon passed the same kind of laws. However, as these laws began to be enforced, opposition started to grow. Often this had a harmful effect, as a number of states repealed the immunization laws. This included California, Illinois, Indiana, Minnesota, Utah, West Virginia, and Wisconsin.

In 1905, in the case *Jacobson v. Massachusetts*, the issue finally came up before the Supreme Court. The court voted to uphold the authority of each state to enforce laws that forced people to get vaccinations. Its reasoning was that this was a case where individual freedom had to be sacrificed for the common good.

In a second Supreme Court case in 1922, the court voted to uphold the right of cities to pass ordinances that required smallpox vaccinations in order to attend school. The people making the case claimed that city ordinances requiring vaccination in order to attend school were a violation of due process and equal protection rights in the Fourteenth Amendment.

This particular case was brought when Rose Zucht, a student in San Antonio, Texas, was not allowed to enroll because she could not show proof of vaccination. The Supreme Court ruled that the claim did not have substance and that legal precedent had established that a) city ordinances were part of state law, and b) state laws requiring vaccination were within the state's power.

2014 MEASLES OUTBREAKS

In 2014, there were 667 cases of measles reported across twenty-seven states. The largest segment of that was a group of 383 cases in Amish communities in Ohio. This cluster was the largest outbreak in the United States since 119 cases were reported in Utah in 1996. The Amish communities, as well as a majority of the other cases, were unvaccinated.

Disneyland

One of these measles outbreaks, in December of 2014, was traced back to Disneyland in Los Angeles and ended up affecting 147 people from seven different states and three different countries. The best theory of the starting point is that it was a traveler from out of the country—likely the Philippines. By the time it wound down, about thirty people had to be hospitalized. The thing that makes this particularly

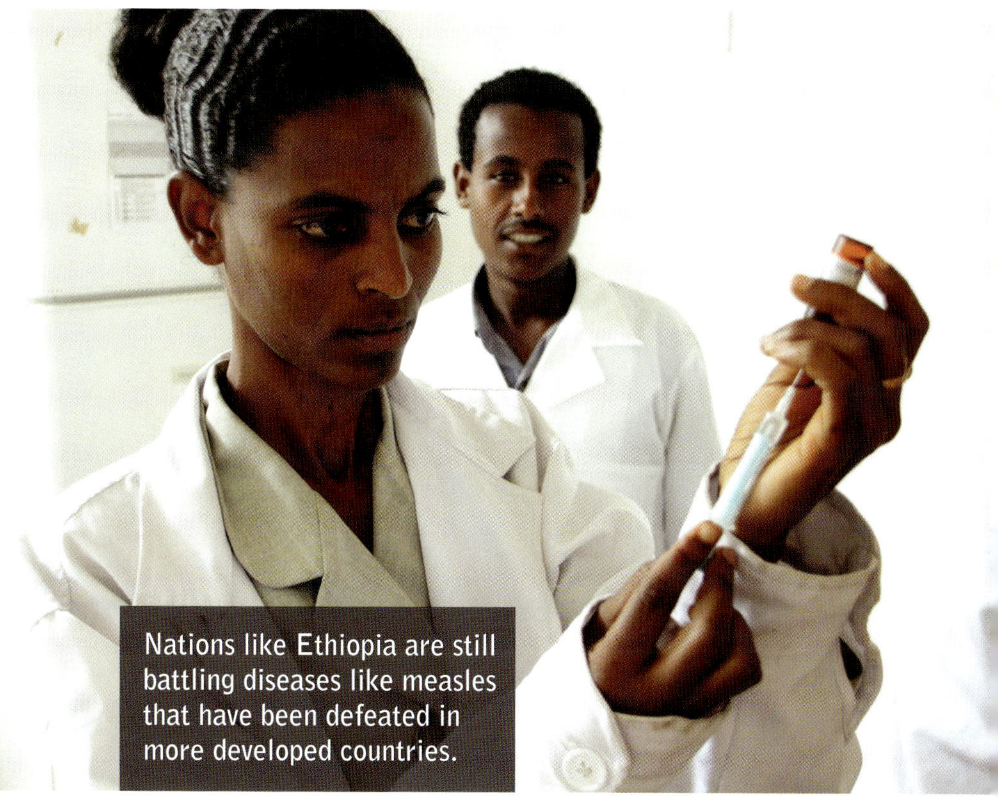
Nations like Ethiopia are still battling diseases like measles that have been defeated in more developed countries.

unsettling is that 92 percent of the people involved did not have their vaccinations.

Then, there was a second outbreak in Quebec, Canada, that started in February of 2015. It was also connected to Disneyland but seems to have been set off by a different initial carrier. Because the members of the religious community it affected had very low vaccination rates, the outbreak spread to 136 people before health officials were able to get a handle on it.

Other Outbreaks

There have also been some smaller outbreaks of measles: one group in Illinois had fifteen, a group in Nevada had nine, and Washington State had a group of five. In all these cases, when officials conducted interviews about not being vaccinated, 43 percent of them claimed it was because of philosophical or religious objections to vaccinations. The others said they were ineligible due to age (too young) or health problems, they had missed opportunities to get vaccinated, and various other reasons.

One of the important issues that came out of this is that some of the children who caught the disease were too young to be vaccinated or had medical issues that prevented them from being able to get vaccinated, so they had been put at risk by the collapse of herd immunity. Basically, they were infected because of someone else's philosophical or religious beliefs or because grown, rational adults couldn't manage to get them their vaccinations. The same is true for a woman in the state of Washington who died because she had been at the health clinic with one of the outbreak patients. Her health issues required her to be on medications that suppress the immune system, so she couldn't be vaccinated.

While many of the cases cited here are about people with religious objections, in the aftermath of these outbreaks, the Center for Disease Control and Prevention (CDC) conducted a national survey. Among those who were still opposed to

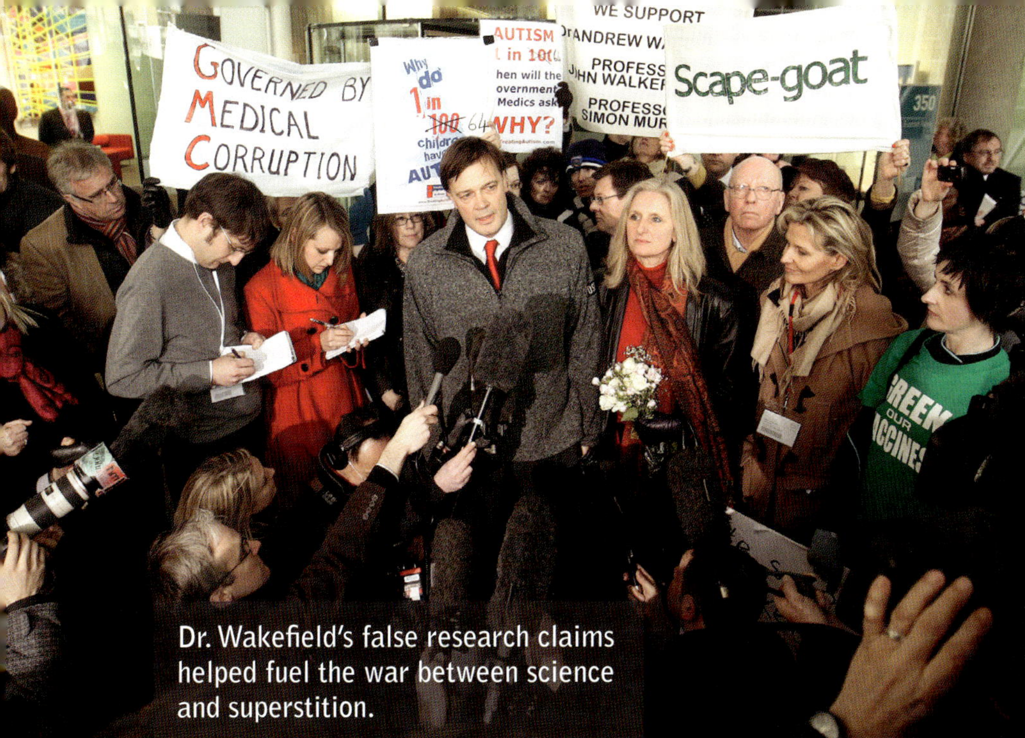

Dr. Wakefield's false research claims helped fuel the war between science and superstition.

having their children vaccinated, the single largest factor was not religious beliefs but fear of side effects of the combined vaccination for measles-mumps-rubella (MMR) and the human papilloma virus (HPV). The dreaded side effects were the various alleged risks, including autism.

FRAUDULENT RESEARCH: GIANT HEADLINES, TINY RETRACTION

One of the major incidents of recent years that helped stoke the fires of fear and resistance against vaccination was the faulty research publicized by Andrew Wakefield. He and some colleagues had a research study published by the British medical journal *Lancet*. In this study, they concluded that the MMR vaccine appeared to cause behavioral problems and developmental disorders in children.

Although the study used only a tiny sample of twelve children to start with, had no control group, and drew sketchy conclusions, it still generated a ton of publicity and was amplified in the popular media. The fear spread among parents, and the rates of vaccinations in England and the United States dropped.

It took six years before ten of the original twelve researchers published a retraction in the *Lancet* saying that there was, in fact, no causal link established in their data. This was compounded by the shady ethics involved, since it turned out that Wakefield was paid a lot of money by lawyers of parents who wanted to sue the drug companies.

Finally, in 2010, after a hearing by the British Medical Council found Wakefield guilty of dishonesty and mistreatment of developmentally challenged children, the *Lancet* published a retraction of the initial article and admitted that Wakefield was guilty of various ethics violations. It is an unfortunate fact that it is much harder to un-scare people than it is to scare them, so even with the retraction and follow-up articles, much of the damage could not be repaired.

An important part of good science is, of course, having others independently test your results. In the years since the scandal, there have been numerous separate research teams that have combed through the records of more than six hundred thousand children. The results have been consistent: the rate of children with autism was the same among children who received the MMR vaccine and those who did not.

There have been even more convincing studies as well. For example, one study looked at almost one hundred thousand children who had high risk factors for developing autism. Even among this very susceptible group, the rate of developing autism after receiving the MMR vaccine was no higher than for children who received the MMR vaccine but did not have high risk factors.

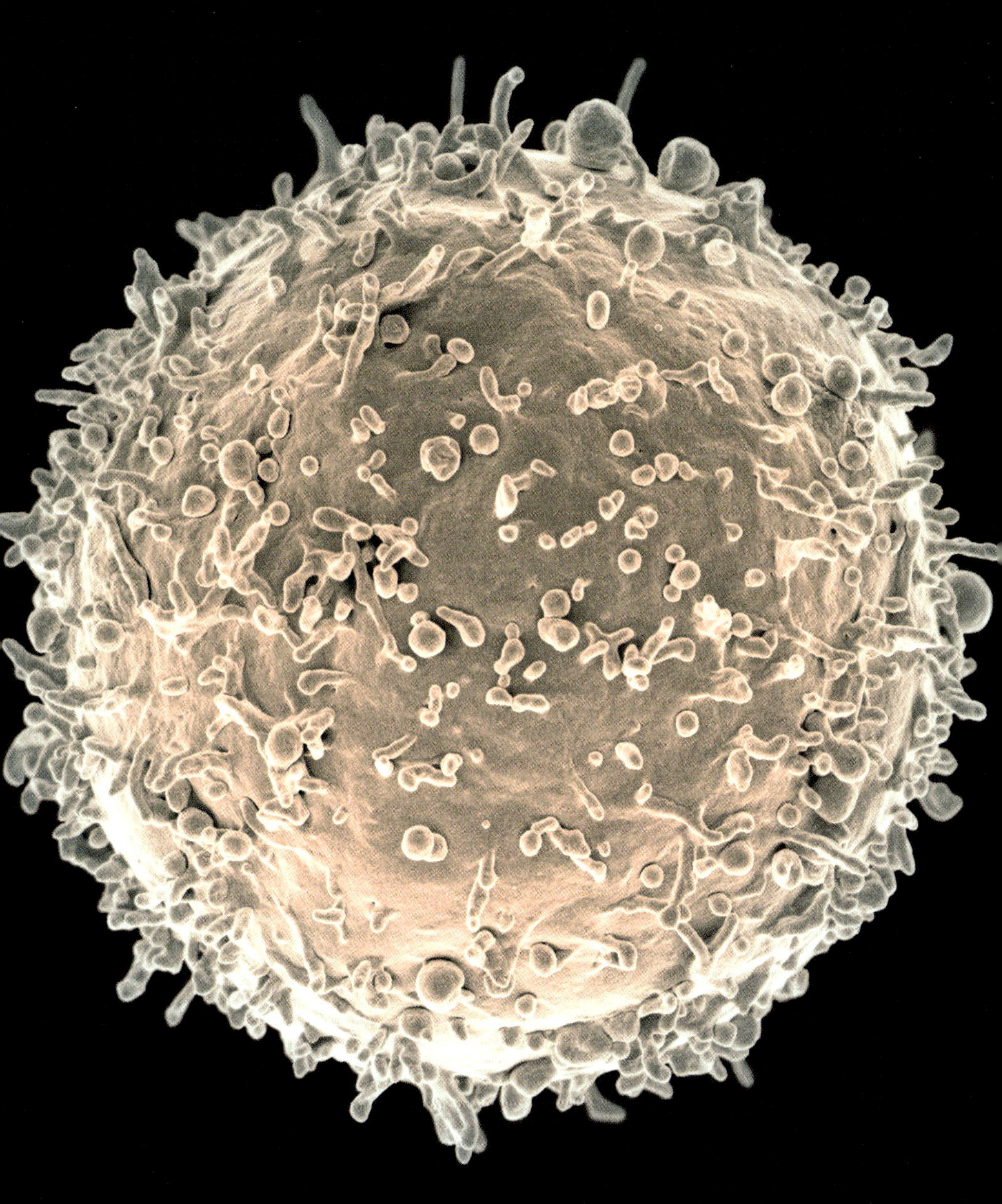

A colorized image of a B-cell
from an electron microscope

The RELIGIOUS RESISTANCE

All the US states have laws that children must have vaccinations in order to attend public school. However, in response to voter pressure, forty-seven of those states allow for exceptions to those rules if the parents have religious objections. California recently repealed these exceptions and no longer allows students to opt out for religious reasons.

Religion and the Battle Against HIV

As we look toward the future of developments in immunology and vaccination, we cannot help but notice that in addition to the normal obstacles of any scientific research, the fight against HIV has at times inspired the same kind of religious thinking that assigned attributed diseases to particular sins.

A survey released in 2014 from the Public Religion Research Institute found that 14 percent of Americans believe AIDS is a punishment from God. There is some slight consolation in that this figure is much lower than the 36 percent who held these beliefs back in 1992.

Sometimes religious policies disarm traditional weapons that are helpful in the fight to contain and combat the spread of contagious diseases. Perhaps none stand out so clearly as the ongoing efforts by the Catholic Church to preach against the use of condoms, which have proven effective in managing the spread of HIV.

FUTURE DIRECTIONS

HIV Strategy: Intermittent Therapy

One of the potentially promising directions of research in battling HIV addresses the problem of outsmarting strains of the virus that mutate to develop resistance to various drugs. The reason this works is because "being resistant" usually costs the virus something in terms of time or energy or resources. Think of it like this: if you are going into battle, you can only carry a certain number of weapons and pieces of equipment. If you pick an extra box of ammunition as one of your items, then either a) you have to leave something else behind—maybe the extra ammo means you can't take your handgun or you can't take as much food or b) you are bogged down with extra weight, which means you are slower, you need more calories to fuel your trip, and so on. Either way, you have made a trade-off that will end up putting you at a disadvantage.

So, let us suppose that a person has HIV and some of the virus is nonresistant strains and some is resistant. Now, if this person has been taking the drug, then there will only be a small population of the nonresistant virus left in his system.

If he stops taking the drug for a time, though, that minority nonresistant population gains the upper hand, killing off the resistant ones. That is, they are faster and have more energy, so they win the competition for resources. At this point, the person is in the reverse situation where the resistant population has been shrunk down to low levels. That means it is time to drop drug bombs into the body to wipe out the nonresistant virus as well.

We have oversimplified somewhat, of course, but it is fascinating to understand this about competition with viruses and to see how a whole new kind of thinking has come into play.

HIV Strategy: Speeding Up Antibody Variation

Another fascinating direction of research in fighting against HIV has to do with ramping up the rate our bodies can produce different varieties of antibodies to be able to catch up to the mutation rate of HIV. Instead of trying to slow down HIV, this strategy works to speed up the immune response.

So, as we discussed, when our bodies encounter an invader, the B-lymphocytes start building antibodies. They do this by putting together building blocks or segments that are known by their letters: D (diversity), J (joining), and V (variable). By putting these together in different combinations and sequences, then, the B-cells can make a wide variety of antibodies.

This is not just a one-round process, though. The B-cells continue tinkering with the sequence and trying new varieties to make the antibodies better and better at fighting that particular invader.

So, researchers have been able to take samples from antibodies that worked for a while or that worked partly against HIV strains (until the viruses mutated around them). They then create mice whose B-cells already have a head start at producing effective combinations for antibodies that might work against HIV. Then when new HIV antigens are introduced, the production of antibodies that work against the new strain already have a kind of head start on how many times the design has to be tinkered with before it works (or so it can keep working).

Part of the real advantage here is that researchers don't have to wait for generation after generation of mice to develop. Instead, they can just switch a certain part of the genetic programming to create new changes in the B-cells that are produced.

HIV Strategy: Speeding Up HIV Mutation

The third strategy that we will cover, as far as HIV goes, uses HIV's own speed against it. As we mentioned, it already reproduces very quickly and the sloppiness builds in a lot of mutations. Professor John Essigmann from the University of Washington and his colleagues are working from the fact that if they can get it to mutate even faster, the result would be so sloppy that it would no longer produce working proteins.

Historic Battles with the Flu

As we looked at with various diseases earlier in the book, here, too, our ability to appreciate the overall risk and impact of the flu comes from a brief timeline of major flu outbreaks.

Still the worst pandemic to date, the Spanish flu outbreak killed between forty million and seventy million people around the world from 1917 to 1918. A great many of these victims died within hours of first falling ill. Interestingly, it started in Kansas but is referred to as the Spanish influenza because it had a particularly devastating impact in Spain during the fall of 1918.

The next flu pandemic was the Asian influenza that struck between 1957 and 1958, discussed earlier. It was followed by the Hong Kong flu in 1968–1969. The death toll was much lower, probably because many people were protected by exposure to the 1957–1958 outbreak. There were approximately thirty-four thousand deaths in the United States and between one and three million around the world.

While the avian flu outbreak that started in 1997 (and is ongoing) spread widely among birds and was transmitted from birds to humans, it never took wing and started moving from human to human. It is still considered a large threat because if it does mutate just enough to transmit among humans, the scale of outbreak will be massive.

Then there is the H1N1 flu virus, which emerged in Mexico in 2009. In the United States, there were estimated to be somewhere between forty-two million and eighty-six million cases, though the relative death rate was lower than previous pandemics, with deaths in America reaching between eight thousand and seventeen thousand.

The Flu: Forward-Thinking Strategies

The point of this separate tour of the history of flu pandemics is to provide a context for why this is an important and ongoing front in the war between humans and viruses. The US Department of Health and Human Services projects that if a pandemic influenza with the strength of the 1918 virus were to ignite, there could be nearly two million US deaths and up to ten million people hospitalized.

It is logical to ask why it is so hard to design a vaccine for a disease like this. One of the key reasons is the flip side of why we were so successful in wiping out smallpox. While smallpox had no place except in humans where it could go to hang out, influenza is quite able to move back and forth between humans and animals. We see this reflected in the names "avian flu," "swine flu," and so on. In order to destroy it, we would have to manage to cure all the cases in people and all the closely related versions in animals all at the same time.

Influenza is not the world champion in mutation speed (that is HIV), but it would be on the medal stand at the Olympics. That also helps to explain why you have to get a new flu shot every year. When you combine that with the last point, you can see that as long as it keeps being able to survive and reproduce, it can adapt to our vaccines.

On top of this, there is a problem of vaccination levels. According to the Health and Human Services website, as of January 2017, the highest vaccination rate was Delaware with 23.98 percent (the lowest was Montana at 11.4 percent, and Washington, DC, coming in second lowest at 11.94 percent). That means not only that many are unprotected, but that we fall below the herd immunity threshold, so infants and the elderly, who are not appropriate patients for the vaccine, are not sheltered, providing the virus ample places to hang out, multiply, and mutate.

A Closer Look at Religious Opposition to Vaccination

As we've seen throughout history, in the twenty-first century some people still interpret their holy scriptures as opposed to vaccination. Two of the most common of these interpretations involve the concepts of contamination and abomination.

The contamination idea argues that we are putting things into our bodies that were not meant to be there according to God's design. Vaccines contain biological by-products, foreign viruses, chemical waste, toxic carcinogens, and animal parts. As a result, by receiving vaccines, some believers think we are doing the equivalent of dumping industrial refuse into our bodies instead of treating them like temples.

Abomination, the other common line of thinking in antivaccination circles, is the argument that we are mixing the blood of animals with human blood, and this goes against God's will in a slightly different way. Because vaccines contain elements of animal blood (serum, antibodies, etc.), this idea holds that we are violating the biblical tenet that human blood is supposed to be kept pure and not mixed with animal blood.

Of course, the vast majority of adherents reconcile science with their biblical beliefs.

Chronology

4000 BCE This is the earliest date of evidence for tuberculosis

430 BCE Athens is decimated by a typhoid epidemic

1514 Andreas Vesalius is born; later, he is the first to develop research based on human dissection

1546 Girolamo Fracastoro's book, *On Contagion*, posits that disease is caused by little particles

1613 Diphtheria levels are so high in Spain it is nicknamed "the Year of Strangulations"

1647 The first outbreak of yellow fever happens in Barbados

1663 Cotton Mather is born

1689 Lady Montagu is born

1717 Lady Montagu sees an inoculation during her time in Turkey

1721 The clergyman Cotton Mather promotes the use of variolation in the United States

1749 Edward Jenner is born

1796 Edward Jenner successfully uses cowpox to inoculate against smallpox

1817 The first of the modern cholera pandemics starts by sweeping across Asia

1822 Louis Pasteur is born

1840 Britain passes the National Vaccine Act

1843 Robert Koch is born

1882 Robert Koch identifies the bacteria that cause tuberculosis

1882 Émile Roux and Alexandre Yersin discover that a vaccine can be developed using toxins instead of a virus

1885 Louis Pasteur successfully tests his rabies vaccine, and production begins

1907 Polio erupts onto the stage, starting with cases in New York

1922 The US Supreme Court upholds the right to make city ordinances for vaccination

1931 Ernst Ruska and his advisor build the first electron microscope, allowing us to see viruses

1954 Jonas Salk's polio vaccine is administered on a wide scale for testing

1980 The World Health Organization declares smallpox eradicated

1981 HIV and AIDS epidemic first breaks out in the United States

2014 There are several measles outbreaks in the United States due to declines in vaccination

Glossary

alchemy A medieval mixture of primitive chemistry and mystical theory; it was partly concerned with chemical transformations (especially turning lead to gold) and partly with a theory of developing human capabilities.

antigens Any toxins or other invading substances that provoke an immune response.

autopsy The careful examination of a body and the internal organs after death.

bacteria Any member of a group of one-celled organisms; many of them cause disease if allowed to enter the body.

charlatans People who pretend or claim to have expertise that they really do not, usually to con people out of their money (especially for a medical process or medication).

cholera A particular type of bacterial infection in the small intestine.

contamination The condition where something harmful or offensive is introduced to a substance, which makes it unsafe to use going forward.

diphtheria A bacterial disease that causes swelling of the mucous membranes as well as heart and nerve damage. A common effect is a thick membrane in the throat that interferes with breathing.

entomologist A person engaged in the scientific study of insects.

epidemics Large outbreaks of an infectious disease.

epidemiology The scientific study of epidemics.

eradication When something has been completely destroyed or eliminated.

extremity In medical contexts, this refers to the arms and legs (especially hands and feet).

fatality A death caused by disease, war, or some sort of accident.

infection Having viruses or bacteria get into the body and begin multiplying.

leprosy An infectious disease that affects nerves, mucous membranes, and the skin. It causes a number of deformities and disfigurements.

lymph glands Another term for lymph nodes. These are small areas in the lymphatic system where lymph (fluid) is filtered and where lymphocytes are formed.

malaria An illness caused when protozoa invade the red blood cells.

measles A contagious viral disease characterized by rash, cough, fever, and sore throat.

metallurgy The branch of science that focuses on the properties of metal, its uses, and the processes of working with it to build things.

miasma A toxic, foul-smelling clump of air. For centuries this was thought to be how disease was communicated.

microbes Any of a variety of tiny organisms, including algae, bacteria, and viruses.

mumps This contagious viral disease causes swelling, fever, and occasionally male sterility.

mutate In biological terms, this refers to the introduction of changes into the DNA sequence of an organism, sometimes adding an advantage and sometimes subtracting some advantage.

outbreak A sudden increase in the number of cases; usually used to describe the spread of diseases.

pandemic An outbreak that has grown and spread to other parts of the world.

pathogens Microbes that can cause disease.

physiology The branch of science dealing with the functions of organisms and their different parts and systems.

polio "Polio" is the common short version of "poliomyelitis." It refers to a viral disease that affects the nervous system, resulting in short-term and long-term paralysis.

protozoa Members of the group of one-celled organisms that live in water or as parasites in another organism.

quarantine The practice of isolating people and animals who have or might have become infected with some contagious disease to help keep it from spreading.

rabies This viral disease affects the brain and nervous system of dogs and other mammals. It can cause convulsions, paralysis, and death. It causes excess saliva and is transmitted from saliva to blood through biting.

replicate To make exact copies; to reproduce.

rubella A contagious viral disease closely related to measles. It used to be referred to as German measles.

serum The pale-yellow fluid part of the blood in which red blood cells and white blood cells are contained; plasma.

smallpox A deadly viral disease characterized by high fevers and pus-filled eruptions on the body that leave scarring.

stigmatization The act of treating someone as unacceptable in normal society, casting him or her out as untouchable for moral disgrace or for medical reasons. In cases like leprosy, it was both.

tetanus This disease is also known as lockjaw. It is a bacterial disease that causes rigidity and powerful spasms of the voluntary muscle system.

toxins Poisons or venoms of plant or animal origin; used especially of those from microorganisms and causing disease.

tuberculosis This infectious bacterial disease is characterized by lumps (called "tubers") in the body, especially the lungs. Particularly deadly because it can become airborne and spread quickly.

variolation The procedure of taking matter (such as pus or scabs) from the wound of a person infected with a disease (like smallpox or cowpox) and using a tool of some kind to put the material into the skin or bloodstream of someone else to stimulate an immune response.

vector An organism that transmits a disease (or a parasite carrying the disease) from one person to another.

virus A microorganism about $1/110^{th}$ the size of bacteria. Its structure is different from an organic cell, and it is only able to reproduce using the cells within another organism.

yellow fever A viral disease common to tropical climates. It creates high fever and affects the kidneys and liver, which can lead to internal bleeding. The yellowish complexion of victims is caused by a buildup of certain compounds in the blood because the liver stops filtering them out.

Further Information

BOOKS

Foege, William H. *House on Fire: The Fight to Eradicate Smallpox*. Berkeley, CA: University of California Press, 2011.

Jacobs, Charlotte DeCroes. *Jonas Salk: A Life*. Oxford, UK: Oxford University Press, 2015.

Oshinsky, David M. *Polio: An American Story*. Oxford, UK: Oxford University Press, 2006.

Youngdahl, Karie, Babi Hammond, and Michelle Sipics. *The History of Vaccines*. Philadelphia, PA: The College of Physicians of Philadelphia, 2013.

WEBSITES

Edward Jenner
https://www.famousscientists.org/edward-anthony-jenner/

Learn more about the life and accomplishments of Edward Jenner.

Guns, Germs, and Steel
http://www.pbs.org/gunsgermssteel/variables/smallpox.html

Read about a number of different topics related to how smallpox shaped history and culture.

The History of Vaccination
https://bigpictureeducation.com/history-vaccination

Explore an overview of the history of vaccines, links to further reading, and comprehension questions.

Microorganisms
http://www.neok12.com/Microorganisms.htm

Take quizzes, watch short videos, and complete other activities on topics related to microorganisms.

The Science Museum
http://www.sciencemuseum.org.uk/broughttolife/themes/science

Learn more about the history of medical science. Explore additional articles about diseases, epidemics, the history of medical theory, and more.

VIDEOS

"Germ Theory"
http://www.sciencechannel.com/tv-shows/greatest-discoveries/videos/100-greatest-discoveries-shorts-germ-theory/

The Science Channel describes a foundational discovery that paved the way for vaccination.

"How Do Vaccines Work? – Kelwalin Dhanasarnsombut"
http://ed.ted.com/lessons/how-do-vaccines-work-kelwalin-dhanasarnsombut

Follow along as this short video traces the history of vaccines and describes the mechanism behind their effectiveness.

"Jonas Salk, M.D.: Developer of the Polio Vaccine"
http://www.achievement.org/achiever/jonas-salk-m-d/#interview

Jonas Salk talks about his big breakthroughs in this inspiring interview.

Bibliography

Aptowitz, Christin O'Keefe. *Dr. Mutter's Marvels: A True Tale of Intrigue and Innovation at the Dawn of Modern Medicine*. New York, NY: Avery, 2015.

Barnard, Bryn. *Outbreak! Plagues That Changed History*. New York, NY: Dragonfly Books, 2015.

Barry, John M. *The Great Influenza: The Story of the Deadliest Pandemic in History*. New York, NY: Penguin Books, 2005.

Biography.com. "Edward Jenner." Retrieved January 1, 2017. http://www.biography.com/people/edward-jenner-9353941.

Bushak, Lecia. "A Brief History of Vaccines: From Medieval Chinese 'Variolation' to Modern Vaccination." Medical Daily, March 21, 2016. http://www.medicaldaily.com/history-vaccines-variolation-378738.

CDC. "Measles Cases and Outbreaks." Retrieved January 1, 2017. https://www.cdc.gov/measles/cases-outbreaks.html.

De Kruif, Paul. *Microbe Hunters*. Boston, MA: Mariner Books, 2002.

Fenn, Elizabeth. *Pox Americana: The Great Smallpox Epidemic of 1775–82*. New York, NY: Hill and Wang, 2002.

Healthy Children. "History of Immunizations." Retrieved January 1, 2017. https://www.healthychildren.org/English/safety-prevention/immunizations/Pages/History-of-Immunizations.aspx.

Heyworth, Kelley King. "Vaccines: The Reality Behind the Debate." *Parents*. Retrieved January 1, 2017. http://www.parents.com/health/vaccines/controversy/vaccines-the-reality-behind-the-debate/.

History of Vaccines. "Different Types of Vaccines." Retrieved January 1, 2017. http://www.historyofvaccines.org/content/articles/different-types-vaccines.

Immunization Advisory Centre. "A Brief History of Vaccines." Retrieved January 1, 2017. http://www.immune.org.nz/brief-history-vaccination.

Jakab, E.A.M. *Louis Pasteur: Hunting Killer Germs*. New York, NY: McGraw-Hill, 2000.

Johnson, Steven. *The Ghost Map: The Story of London's Most Terrifying Epidemic—and How It Changed Science, Cities, and the Modern World*. New York, NY: Riverhead, 2007.

Klein, Christopher. "8 Things You May Not Know About Jonas Salk and the Polio Vaccine." History Channel, October 28, 2014. http://www.history.com/news/8-things-you-may-not-know-about-jonas-salk-and-the-polio-vaccine.

Marrin, Albert. *Dr. Jenner and the Speckled Monster: The Discovery of the Smallpox Vaccine*. New York NY: Dutton, 2002.

Matthews, Robert. "Lady Montagu's Daring Cure (It Only Killed One in Eight)." *Telegraph*, April 5, 2001. http://www.telegraph.co.uk/news/science/science-news/4761718/Lady-Marys-daring-cure-it-only-killed-one-in-eight.html.

Mayo Clinic. "Mumps." Retrieved January 1, 2017. http://www.mayoclinic.org/diseases-conditions/mumps/basics/definition/con-20019914.

McNeil, William H. *Plagues and People*. New York, NY: Anchor, 1976.

Montagu, Lady Mary Wortley. *Turkish Embassy Letters*. Edited by Jack Malcolm. New York, NY: Virago, 1994.

Murphy, Jim. *An American Plague: The True and Terrifying Story of the Yellow Fever Epidemic of 1793*. Boston, MA: Clarion Books, 2003.

NBC News. "Measles Outbreak Traced to Disneyland Is Declared Over." April 17, 2015. http://www.nbcnews.com/storyline/measles-outbreak/measles-outbreak-traced-disneyland-declared-over-n343686.

NHS. "The History of Vaccines." Retrieved January 1, 2017. http://www.nhs.uk/Conditions/vaccinations/Pages/the-history-of-vaccination.aspx.

Oldstone, Michael B. A. *Viruses, Plagues, and History: Past, Present and Future*. Oxford, UK: Oxford University Press, 2006.

Otto, Shawn. *The War on Science: Who's Waging It, Why It Matters, and What We Can Do About It*. Minneapolis, MN: Milkweed Editions, 2016.

Parks, Peggy. *Giants of Science—Jonas Salk*. Woodbridge, CT: Blackbirch Marketing, 2003.

PBS. "Jonas Salk." Retrieved Jauary 1, 2017. http://www.pbs.org/wgbh/aso/databank/entries/bmsalk.html.

Roosink, Marilyn J. *Virus: An Illustrated Guide to 101 Incredible Microbes*. Princeton, NJ: Princeton University Press, 2016.

Rosenberg, Charles E. *The Cholera Years: The United States in 1832, 1849, and 1866*. Chicago, IL: University of Chicago Press, 1987.

Salk Institute for Biological Studies. "About Salk." Retrieved January 1, 2017. http://www.salk.edu/about/history-of-salk/jonas-salk/.

Wasik, Bill, and Monica Murphy. *Rabid: A Cultural History of the World's Most Diabolical Virus*. New York, NY: Viking, 2012.

World Health Organization. "History of Vaccine Development." Retrieved January 1, 2017. http://vaccine-safety-training.org/history-of-vaccine-development.html.

Yong, Edward. *I Contain Multitudes: The Microbes Within Us and a Grander View of Life*. New York, NY: Ecco, 2016.

Zimmer, Carl. *A Planet of Viruses: 2nd Edition*. Chicago IL: University of Chicago Press, 2015.

Index

Page numbers in **boldface** are illustrations. Entries in **boldface** are glossary terms.

About the Author

Erik Richardson is an award-winning teacher from Milwaukee. While he is on sabbatical from teaching middle school math and science, he is teaching a variety of college courses. In addition to writing in his free time, he also runs a small nonprofit called Every Einstein that works to provide STEM resources for students and teachers around the country.